# TARGETING IN MENTAL HEALTH SERVICES

*For Rob*

*and*

*For Margaret, Dyfan, Iestyn and Bethan*

# Targeting in Mental Health Services
## A multi-disciplinary challenge

*Edited by*

**LESLEY COTTERILL**
*Department of Sociology*
*University of Plymouth*

**WALLY BARR**
*Health and Community Care Research Unit*
*University of Liverpool*

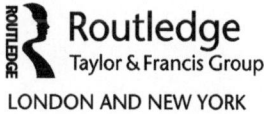

Routledge
Taylor & Francis Group

LONDON AND NEW YORK

First published 2000 by Ashgate Publishing

Reissued 2019 by Routledge
2 Park Square, Milton Park, Abingdon, Oxon, OX1 4 4RN
52 Vanderbilt Avenue, New York, NY 10017

*Routledge is an imprint of the Taylor & Francis Group, an informa business*

Publisher's Note
The publisher has gone to great lengths to ensure the quality of this reprint but points out that some imperfections in the original copies may be apparent.

Disclaimer
The publisher has made every effort to trace copyright holders and welcomes correspondence from those they have been unable to contact.

A Library of Congress record exists under LC control number:

ISBN 13: 978-1-138-72413-6 (hbk)
ISBN 13: 978-1-138-72411-2 (pbk)
ISBN 13: 978-1-315-19262-8 (ebk)

# Contents

# List of Figures

# List of Tables

# List of Contributors

Dr Mark Agius (MD)
Medical Adviser
Bedfordshire and Luton Community NHS Trust
Luton

Dr Wally Barr (BSc, MA, PhD, RMN, CQSW)
Research Fellow
Health and Community Care Research Unit
University of Liverpool
Liverpool

John Butler (BSC, MSc, FAETC, RMN, Cert. Couns)
CMHC Manager, LeadCMHN, Practice Facilitator
Bedfordshire and Luton Community NHS Trust
Luton

Maggie Clifton (BA, MA, Cert.Man)
Research and Clinical Effectiveness Co-ordinator
Ashworth Hospital Authority
Merseyside

Dr Lesley Cotterill (BA, PhD)
Senior Lecturer/ Evaluation Advisor Plymouth HAZ
University of Plymouth
Plymouth

Dr Ian Davidson (MB, ChB, MRCPsych)
Consultant Psychiatrist/ Clinical Director
Wirral and West Cheshire Community NHS Trust
Chester

David Duffy (BA, MSc, Cert.HSM, RMN)
Professional Head of Nursing
Mental Health Services of Salford NHS Trust
Salford

Dr Robert Wyn Edwards (MB, Ch.B, DRCOG)
GP Principal
Vittoria Medical Centre
Birkenhead
Merseyside

Sara Finlayson (BSc Hons, MPhil, DipClinPsychol)
Clinical Psychologist
Rathbone Hospital HDU
Liverpool

Paul Golding
Welfare Benefits Specialist
Wallasey CAB
Merseyside

Dr Ann Hoskins (MB, BcH, BAO, Mcomm.H, FFPHM)
Director of Public Health
Manchester Health Authority
Manchester

Professor Peter Huxley (PhD, CQSW)
Professor of Social Work
Health Services Research Department
(Social Work and Social Care Section)
Institute of Psychiatry
King's College
London

Gary Lees (BSc, MA, Dip. HSM, RMN)
Lead CMHN/ Clinical Development
Bedfordshire and Luton Community NHS Trust
Luton

Mick McKeown (BA Hons, RGN, RMN, DPSN Thorn)
Principal Lecturer (Mental Health Nursing Research)
Department of Primary and Community Nursing
University of Central Lancashire
Preston

Dave Mercer (BA Hons, MA, RMN, PGCE)
Lecturer
Department of Nursing
University of Liverpool
Liverpool

Gurch Randhawa (BSc, MSc)
Principal Lecturer
Institute for Health Services Research
University of Luton
Luton

Siobhan Reilly (BSc)
Research and Development Officer
Dementia Centre
PSSRU
Department of Psychiatry
University of Manchester
Manchester

Eva Robinshaw (BA)
Research Associate
Mental Health Social Work Research Unit
Department of Psychiatry
University of Manchester
Manchester

Dr Vimal Kumar Sharma (MBBS, MD, PhD, FRCPsych.)
Consultant Psychiatrist and Honorary Senior Lecturer
Wirral and West Cheshire Community NHS Trust/University of Liverpool
Merseyside

William Spence (BSc, MEd, RMN, DipPSN)
Principal Lecturer
Department of Public and Community Health
Oxford Brookes University
Oxford

Helen Sumner (BSocSc, MA, CQSW)
Assistant Director Special Needs and Disability
Warrington Social Services
Warrington

Robin Williams (MSc, RMN, SRN, CPN Cert, Dip.Nursing, Dip. IHSM)
Nurse Clinician
St Hilary Brow Group Practice
Wallasey

# PART 1
# SETTING THE SCENE

# Introduction

This book has its origins in a three-year research project initially entitled 'Do SEMI Registers Make a Difference?' and known, for short, as the *SEMI Registers Project*. The research project was designed to monitor and evaluate the introduction of registers for people with severe and enduring mental illness (SEMI) in general practices across the Wirral. The project was action-oriented, with feedback channelled through an Advisory Group. The first phase of the project involved monitoring the implementation process. The second phase, from which the project got its name, involved an evaluation of the extent to which introducing these registers made a positive difference to the quality of care and quality of life experienced by people with SEMI who were included on these registers.

The plan to introduce SEMI registers, the *SEMI Registers Initiative*, was part of Wirral's Mental Health Strategy. The decision to have the SEMI Registers project run in parallel to the initiative was taken forward by Ann Hoskins, then Director of Public Health in the Wirral, who wrote the first draft of the proposal for research funding. Then, the editors of this book became involved in the further development of the proposal, and subsequently became the research team based at the Health and Community Care Research Unit, University of Liverpool.

At the start of the research project, we traced the idea of targeting people with SEMI in policy and practice, and began to reflect on the utility of the idea, how this goal might best be achieved, and the sorts of concerns associated with it. We began to ask ourselves questions about targeting that we regarded as pre-requisites to the targeting agenda. These questions included: How is the term 'severe and enduring mental illness' to be defined? By what method are people with SEMI to be identified and targeted? With what are they to be targeted, and by whom? Most importantly, what is the expected effect of such targeting, and what will be the outcomes in the short, medium and long-term? How will such initiatives be evaluated, and from whose perspective? What are the associated problems, or unintended consequences? And so the list went on. Our involvement in the SEMI Registers Project gave us the chance to explore these questions and gain some insight into the extent to which they were being addressed in one particular study. This book gives another opportunity to develop and extend these lines of inquiry.

As the research project progressed, the preliminary findings from the first phase of the project alerted us to the corollary of issues surrounding the notion of targeting, in the context of setting up SEMI registers. These issues include the social, ethical, political, sociological, legal and practical dimensions of the enterprise. Consideration of these issues highlighted the need for conceptual analysis, policy evaluation and theory building in this area. Our personal experience of the research process underlined the appropriateness of the action-oriented approach, and raised our awareness of the local political context within which the Registers Initiative was being introduced. At national level, the social and political context is now dominated by the government's mental health modernisation agenda.

Reviewing the literature for the SEMI Registers project revealed that, since their inception, community mental health nurses (CPNs) were expected to cater for many of the needs of people with SEMI. Despite this intention, successive research projects (with some exceptions) reported that this was not happening in many areas. In contrast, people with less severe mental health problems, dubbed 'the worried well', were found to be filling CPN case loads, with little time, and some suggested little enthusiasm, left for working with people with SEMI. In the 1990s, the trends towards developing a primary care-led NHS influenced the tendency for CPNs to become 'attached to', or located within, GP surgeries. This shift in location increasingly resulted in CPNs becoming more greatly involved in counselling and other activities appropriate for the needs of many of the people with mental health problems presenting in primary care settings. During the same period, the well-publicised series of incidents involving people with SEMI in acts of violence led to rising public concern, and highlighted the failures in care experienced by people with SEMI. The government's pressing need to be seen to act in response to this state of affairs resulted in the introduction of a variety of policy developments and initiatives designed to 'close the gap' in the 'net of care'. Some have argued that these developments (e.g. Supervision Registers and the power of supervised discharge) heralded the beginning of a more coercive, socially controlling era in mental health care. Indeed, prior to the introduction of several measures and initiatives during the early 1990s, academics and practitioners alike declared key components of the government's plan to be flawed. This was a cause of some concern, given that such measures were intended to effectively manage the risk posed by some people with SEMI in the community.

More recently, the New Labour administration has announced its health and social care modernisation programme and, within that, the proposed mental health reforms. Implementation is currently ongoing. The mental health reforms have the backing of extra funding, a commitment to improve quality and raise standards, and to deliver comprehensive mental health services that are informed by research evidence and best practice. These changes are to be monitored by new structures to deliver effective performance assessment and management. Alongside quality improvement, safety is now the main priority in mental health services, and targeting people with SEMI for specialist intervention is a cornerstone of the strategy to achieve this goal. The continuation of the trend in targeting people with SEMI for specialist intervention has the support of a national service framework and proposed changes to mental health legislation.

In the context of this discussion, and within the framework of the mental health and social care reforms currently being introduced, key issues in the targeting agenda include:

- definitional issues surrounding the term 'SEMI';
- practical and methodological concerns about how people with SEMI are to be identified and targeted;
- interface issues relating to multi-disciplinary working between primary and secondary care;
- issues concerning the evidence-base for risk management policies and strategies;
- the role of training in effective targeting;
- reflection on the potential consequences of targeting policies and initiatives; and,
- the meaningful involvement of service users from all sections of society.

Additionally, the policy directive to target people with SEMI warrants further scrutiny in order to 'unpack' some of the implicit assumptions by which it is under-pinned. According to the received wisdom of successive administrations, the strategy appears to be a rational approach: scarce resources should be targeted on people with the greatest needs. This has face validity in terms of the drive towards improving efficiency and cost-effectiveness within public services. However, the implicit assumptions that require serious consideration include the notions that:

- people with SEMI can be accurately and consistently identified;
- people with SEMI have the greatest mental health needs;
- meeting those needs will roughly equate with effective risk management;

- resources are scarce and finite; and,
- the strategy does not have any negative, unintended consequences.

These issues and assumptions are examined further in this book and serve as unifying themes for the contributed chapters. In some chapters, a particular issue may be the focus of a piece of research, or an initiative. In others, one or more issues are examined from different perspectives.

The contributors to this edited collection are drawn from different disciplinary, professional and practice backgrounds, bringing the benefit of their insights and experience to bear on the challenge presented by the mental health policy directive to target people with SEMI. The backgrounds of the authors, therefore, reflect the multi-disciplinary nature of the challenge before them, of working in partnership to deliver the government's promise of 'safe, sound and supportive' mental health services.

The book is divided into four sections. The first section, 'Setting the Scene', is comprised of three very different types of chapter, each of which begins the process of sketching-in the background for what is to follow. Chapter 1, by Lesley Cotterill and Wally Barr provides a descriptive account of the policy framework for the modernisation of mental health services. In this chapter, mental health policy is located in the context of the wider health and social care modernisation programme because of the common structures relating to quality improvement, the shift towards a primary care-led NHS, the public health agenda, and the focus on partnership working. In addition, the chapter traces the emergence of the trend towards targeting people with SEMI in policy and practice over the last decade. The chapter ends with some brief comments about the government's prioritisation of safety in its mental health reforms, and the tension this poses for the stated commitment to reducing discrimination.

In chapter 2, Maggie Clifton and David Duffy address the theme of safety in mental health services through the recommendations of mental health inquiry reports. They begin with a brief critique of the inquiry system before presenting the findings of a research project that collated and analysed the recommendations contained in 42 mental health inquiry reports published in the 1990s. In view of the priority the government attaches to improving safety and quality in its mental health services, this important piece of work represents an obvious starting point in understanding the failures of the past, and a means to prevent similar failures in the future. However, despite the status attached to these inquiries and, with one or two exceptions, this type of analysis has been largely absent from the academic and practitioner literature. This omission is wasteful of public resources in that it precludes effective dissemination of such recommendations to inform policy and practice.

The final chapter in this section, by William Spence, presents a medical sociological analysis of the phenomenon of targeting people with 'serious mental illness'. In this chapter, William focuses on the role of language in shaping our understanding of psychiatric terminology, and applies the concept of 'moral panic' to the directive to target people with this identifier for specialist intervention. This chapter is intended to provoke thought about the received wisdom and taken-for-granted assumptions that form the staple diet of much of the policy, and some of the practice, relating to people with SEMI. Whilst the 'medical model' has different connotations for different people, the reality of much funded research is that it is dominated by this broad world-view. However, by virtue of its place within the opening section, this chapter challenges the orthodoxy of the medical model of 'severe mental illness', and serves as something of an 'antidote' to the implicit assumptions that some of the remaining chapters may be accused of containing. In addition, the chapter also challenges the political motive behind the public safety orientation of mental health policy and, to that extent, counters the tendency of the chapter on the policy context to present an 'evolutionary account' of policy formation.

In section two, a selection of opinion-based chapters written from different stakeholder perspectives is presented. No claims are made for this being comprehensive in terms of the coverage of key stakeholder perspectives. Furthermore, the chapters make no pretensions to be *the* perspective of psychiatrists or of social services staff, and so on. As their titles imply, they represent 'a' perspective written from a particular vantage-point in the mental health and social care system. The authors creatively reflect on their personal and professional experience to begin the process of thinking through the import of the targeting directive, and focusing on key issues to be addressed in the implementation of the mental health reforms.

In the first chapter in this section, Ian Davidson 'unpacks' the notion of targeting and explores several key dimensions of the enterprise, including the advantages and disadvantages. The points he raises warrant careful consideration at whatever level one may be involved in targeting people with SEMI. Targeting, Ian argues, is inevitable and will be shaped by the various policy developments contained in the mental health reforms. At its best, targeting will prompt active questioning and goal setting. It is most likely to be beneficial when there is clarity about what is to be achieved, coupled with on-going monitoring and evaluation linked to the various costs, benefits and outcomes. The importance of training is emphasised in the concluding discussion, a theme continued in section 4 by Mick McKeown and colleagues, and by Mark Agius and John Butler.

In chapter 5, Helen Sumner examines the connotations of targeting and the implications of this policy directive. She discusses the challenges facing social workers and social care in identifying an appropriate response, and explores some possible, unintended consequences and conflicting demands implicit in targeting. Helen highlights the inter-dependence of health and social services, recognising that targeting in health can affect decision-making in social care, and vice versa. She also draws attention to the research conducted by Peter Huxley and colleagues into the care provided by health and social services for people with severe mental illness. This topic is addressed in section 3, chapter 9. Helen suggests a possible way forward for health and social care agencies through greater clarification of the responsibility of statutory providers, and a creative approach to supporting and encouraging the development of informal care in the community.

In chapter 6, Bob Edwards provides a GP's perspective on targeting based on his involvement in setting up a SEMI register in the practice where he works. This chapter relates to the Registers Initiative described above, and is the first of three chapters in this edited collection to focus specifically on an aspect of SEMI registers. The chapter begins with an examination of the recent history of managing people with SEMI in the primary care setting, and goes on to explore some of the issues and conflicts which have arisen since the establishment of a practice SEMI register. Later in the book, Wally Barr and Lesley Cotterill report findings from the SEMI Registers Project, and Robin Williams presents a detailed account of how to set up a practice-based register.

Paul Golding, who gives his opinions on targeting people with SEMI from a service user's perspective, writes the final chapter in this section. He draws on his experience as an advocate, an advice worker and representative of a Mental Health Forum to explore some contentious issues in mental health policy and practice, especially the fate of people with SEMI living in the community. Paul focuses on the themes of stigma and discrimination, the relationship between power and treatment, and the current focus on public health and primary care. He argues that people with SEMI are increasingly singled out for greater social control measures, and urges us to call a halt to the situation where we, as a society, continue to fail the people we espouse to protect and empower.

The third section of the book contains examples of research on discrete but related aspects of targeting people with SEMI. All three chapters are concerned with defining and identifying people with SEMI, chapters 8 and 10 in relation to primary care, and chapter 9 the health and social care interface. The first chapter in this section, by Ann Hoskins, describes a research study that explored the needs of primary care patients who met the criteria for 'severe enduring mental illness'. The study was based in an English health district and collected data from several representative general practices. These data provided a measure of the prevalence of severe enduring mental illness in the practice populations, and an assessment of the use of primary care and secondary mental health services by people with severe enduring mental illness.

Chapter 9 is based on a project funded by the Department of Health, which was designed to establish rates of severe mental illness in  users of health and social services in a number of geographical locations. In this chapter, Peter Huxley, Siobhan Reilly and Eva Robinshaw describe the development of a novel approach to the problem of defining 'severe mental illness'. The approach has the advantage over previous definitions of being based on a continuous rather than a categorical scale. This allows the threshold for meeting the criteria of 'severe mental illness' to be varied according to local circumstances. The authors go on to present the results of a comparison of the characteristics of severely mentally ill service users in contact with either health or social services. These findings highlight similarities and differences in service users and raise a number of questions about the logic of providing care for people with severe mental illness from the two separate agencies.

In chapter 10, Wally Barr and Lesley Cotterill describe the SEMI Registers project that was the catalyst behind this edited collection. The chapter begins with an outline of the thinking behind the introduction of the initiative to establish mental health registers in all general practices across the Wirral. The registers were intended to hold details of practice patients with severe and enduring mental illness and were each kept within the relevant practice. As part of Wirral's 'Mental Health Strategy', there were ambitious aims attached to this initiative surrounding anticipated changes to the co-ordination and quality of care received by people with SEMI, and associated changes to their quality of life in the community. The SEMI Registers project was a three-year study to monitor the process of setting-up the SEMI registers, and evaluate the effects of registration on both patients and carers. Preliminary research findings are presented which highlight some of the pitfalls in implementing this initiative, and this is accompanied by a discussion of the implications of the findings for both practitioners and future research.

The final section contains a selection of initiatives relevant to targeting people with SEMI for specialist intervention. The chapters vary in scope and specificity. The first chapter in this section, written by Gurch Randhawa, focuses on targeting people with SEMI from minority ethnic communities. The chapter begins with a review of the literature concerning ethnicity and mental health as the background context to the 'Partnerships for Change' initiative in Bedfordshire. This initiative aimed to identify the pre-requisites and components of culturally competent mental health services. Findings from the initiative are presented which suggest that discrete initiatives are unlikely to secure the changes needed to address the issue of inequality of access to mental health services for this section of the community, or to result in the provision of culturally competent mental health services. Gurch concludes that to effectively target people with SEMI from ethnic minority communities, issues identified in the literature and the initiative need to become part of the mainstream NHS agenda.

In chapter 12, Mick McKeown, Dave Mercer and Sara Finlayson examine the role of training in the targeting agenda. The chapter begins with a critical appraisal of the mental health inquiry system and a discussion of risk and its management through the use of psychosocial interventions. The authors describe leading-edge training programmes designed to transform service provision through equipping trainees with specialist skills that are then taken back to service settings for wider dissemination. They review the success of these programmes to date, and highlight the lack of attention to the training needs of practitioners working in in-patient services. Against this background, the authors describe a training initiative delivered in Liverpool which they term 'organic training'. The innovative feature of this model concerns the 'whole team' approach to the training enterprise, together with the 'in house' location of the scheme. Initial assessment suggests this approach has much to offer.

The next three chapters focus mainly on primary care in targeting people with SEMI. Two of the chapters address issues at the interface between primary and secondary care. Both of these foci are appropriate in the light of the health and social care reforms that introduce an expanded role for primary care, and emphasise partnership working. Mark Agius and John Butler write the first of these chapters in which they describe an educational initiative designed to meet the needs of primary health care teams in South Bedfordshire. The initiative has been awarded NHS beacon status. The chapter begins with a brief discussion of the need to educate the primary health care team about various aspects of mental illness and its management in primary care. The educational initiative aims to meet these identified needs and to enhance the management of mental health care at the interface between primary care and secondary mental health services through the provision of training in topics such as risk assessment and the use of specialist interventions. The authors describe the development and delivery of the initiative, which resulted in the production of a range of packages and workshops containing information and guidelines about common mental health problems and their management.

In chapter 14, Vimal Sharma focuses on the important topic of effective team-working at the interface between primary and secondary mental health services. The chapter is based on the author's experiences of the 'Primary Care Mental Health Project' in Liverpool. The chapter begins with a discussion of the importance of multi-disciplinary team working in the provision of community-based mental health services, and the barriers to achieving this. Vimal goes on to outline the components of successful team working in the care of people with severe mental illness, and describes the process, problems and benefits of establishing an effective mental health team in a primary care setting in Liverpool.

The next chapter, by Robin Williams, concerns a different, but related, aspect of the effective management of mental health in primary care. Robin provides a detailed description of the procedure adopted by one general practice in setting-up a register of all patients with SEMI. The practice has also taken the route of providing a wide range of mental health services from within the primary care setting. When this approach is taken in conjunction with the proactive use of the mental health register, practice staff are confident that it demonstrates the feasibility and benefits of providing most mental health care from within the practice.

The final chapter, by John Butler and Gary Lees, concerns effective risk assessment and risk management by community mental health nurses. The chapter begins with a detailed account of the definition and identification of risk. Against this background, the authors introduce the 'South Bedfordshire Initiative' in which they were involved. The aim of this initiative was to produce a practical guide for use by community mental health nurses. John and Gary draw on their clinical experience to illustrate the application of theory and practice guidelines to real life situations presented in the form of case study vignettes. The chapter concludes by discussing key features of the management plan.

Neither a discussion, nor tentative comments about 'the way forward' conclude this edited collection. This is quite deliberate and is based on the recognition that this book is an initial exploration of the policy directive to target people with SEMI. More chapters could have been added, but the additional gain would have likely been a diminishing one. 'The way forward' will depend on how the raft of policies designed to transform mental health services over the coming years is implemented, or not. The extent to which the government can be judged to have successfully achieved its stated aims in respect of improving the quality, safety and comprehensiveness of its mental health services awaits future assessment and evaluation.

Lesley Cotterill and Wally Barr
February 2000

# 1 Targeting in Mental Health Services: The Policy Context

LESLEY COTTERILL AND WALLY BARR

## Introduction

Community care for people with mental health problems has a long history spanning several decades. During that time, there has been continuous criticism about the lack of progress towards policy goals. The introduction of the *NHS and Community Care Act* (House of Commons, 1990) breathed new life into old debates about the way forward for mental health services, and gave hope to many that the political will existed to make it a success. However, implementing the policy was delayed until 1993, and thereafter progress was variable across the country. Also, the 1990s were punctuated by a series of highly publicised incidents involving people with mental illness in acts of violence. The subsequent inquiry reports pointed to a host of failings in service provision, especially for people with severe and enduring mental illness (SEMI). In response to the perceived public concern, the government of the day announced various initiatives that were designed to close the gaps in the 'net of care' and improve risk management. These initiatives were characterised by a tendency to be overly legalistic; to introduce a greater element of coercion into practice; to target people with SEMI; and, to have no extra resources attached to the proposals (e.g. DoH, 1994a; House of Commons, 1996).

As we enter the 21$^{st}$ century, the development of mental health services is subject to the changes associated with new Labour's health and social care reforms. The reforms are part of a comprehensive modernisation programme, in which policies are inter-linked to provide 'joined up' solutions to problems, rather than attempt to tamper with parts of the system, or issues in isolation. Recurrent themes within the raft of policy documents include improving the health of the population, reducing health inequalities, and improving quality in service provision. These concerns stem from the identification of unacceptable variations in health, and in the efficiency and effectiveness of health care, across the country. New Labour propose a 'third way' in health and social care which they term 'integrated care' (DoH, 1997a). Integrated care is contrasted with previous policy and practice in that it is intended to be 'based on partnership and driven by performance' (*ibid*, section 2.2), thereby replacing competition with co-operation. In order to emphasise partnership working, the government issued joint priorities guidance to health and social services and, within this circular, identified mental health as a national priority (DoH, 1998a).

The policy context for mental health is 'dove-tailed' into the health and social care reforms, with additional emphasis placed on 'safety', and the involvement of the specialist, secondary services. The concern with 'safety' is rooted in the shortcomings of the mental health services and the continued focus on individual examples of system failure. The government's vision of a 'third way' in mental health involves a modernisation programme to deliver 'safe, sound and supportive' mental health services backed by investment, national standards and legislative reform (DoH, 1998b; 1999a; 1999b). This vision is based on an assessment of community care as a poorly implemented and flawed policy that has failed a significant minority of people, and destroyed the confidence of the general public.

This chapter will begin with an overview of the broad range of health and social care reforms introduced by New Labour and detailed in their key policy documents. Then, under the heading of 'improving quality', a description will be given of the major developments and changes introduced by these policies. The theme of improving quality has been chosen because of its centrality to the overall goals of the modernisation programme, and because of the links between the structures, systems and initiatives designed to deliver this policy goal. However, as these policy documents are inter-linked, there is inevitably some repetition in descriptions of parallel structures and initiatives. For this reason, many of the changes discussed will be referenced to one key document, although they are mentioned in others. This account of the health and social care modernisation programme will provide the background context for the description of the reform and modernisation of mental health services.

Next, because of its relevance to the goal of ensuring safety in mental health practice, and because it forms one of the main planks of the government's mental health strategy, the theme of targeting people with SEMI will be located in policy. The chapter concludes with a brief discussion of some of the issues and contradictions, at the level of policy, raised in this account of the policy context for the development of mental health services.

**The Health and Social Care Reforms**

During the late 1990s, the New Labour government set out its proposals to modernise health and social care in a comprehensive range of policy documents (DoH, 1997a; 1998c; 1998d; 1998e; 1998f; 1999c; 1999d; House of Commons, 1999). In the NHS White Paper, *The New NHS* (DoH, 1997a) the government announced that it intended to build a health service that is 'fit for the twenty-first century'. This is described as:

> A National Health Service which offers people prompt high quality treatment and care when and where they need it. An NHS that does not just treat people when they are ill but works with others to improve health and reduce health inequalities (*ibid.*, section 1.1).

The principles that underpin the proposed reforms involve:

- renewing the NHS as a national service;
- making the delivery of healthcare against national standards a local responsibility;
- encouraging partnership working to produce patient-centred care;
- delivering efficiency gains through rigorous performance management;
- focusing on quality of care to guarantee excellence of service to patients; and
- rebuilding public confidence (*ibid.*, see section 2.4).

The government introduced a ten-year modernisation programme for health and social care services, with investment of £18 billion for the NHS and £3 billion for social services over the next three years. This Modernisation Fund was established to reform and rebuild the NHS. Over the next three years, £5 billion of this money is intended to fund developments designed to improve services including:

- cutting waiting lists;
- modernising hospitals and systems;
- investing in NHS staff;
- ensuring safe and effective mental health care;
- providing better primary care; and,
- improving health promotion (DoH, 1998c, see section 7.6).

The 'third way' for the NHS is to be one that is 'committed to building on what has worked, but discarding what has failed,' (DoH, 1997a, section 2.1). 'What has worked' refers especially to keeping the separation between the planning and provision of hospital services, and to the role of primary care in the commissioning of services, thus aligning clinical and financial responsibility. 'What has failed' refers mainly to the internal market, which is blamed for fostering competition, inefficiency, bureaucracy, secrecy, and producing fragmentation in service provision.

The government's vision is based on an analysis of the problems associated with the internal market (see Table 1.1). The internal market is to be abolished in favour of a system of 'integrated care'. *The New NHS* (DoH, 1997a) outlined plans for far-reaching changes in primary care, with the establishment of primary care groups (PCGs) and, subsequently, primary care trusts (PCTs). In addition, changes to the law relating to primary care were introduced in the *Health Act* (House of Commons, 1999) to facilitate innovation in the organisation and delivery of services. In each area, PCGs bring together GPs and community nurses. The purpose is to promote the health of local people, contributing to the health improvement programmes (HIPs); commissioning health services for the local population from NHS Trusts (within the framework of the HIP); monitoring performance; and, developing primary care through joint working. In order to ensure that national targets will be delivered in each local authority, health authorities have been set the task of agreeing and setting targets with PCGs who, in turn, will develop service agreements with NHS Trusts. In addition, PCG/Ts and NHS Trusts have been given a duty of quality to be discharged through clinical governance. These developments will be discussed in more detail below.

The government's commitment to cut waiting lists is complemented by developments in three key locations:

- at home: easier and faster advice and information for people about health, illness and the NHS;
- in the community: swift advice and treatment in local surgeries and health centres; and,
- in hospital: prompt access to specialist services (DoH, 1997a, see section 1.7).

**Table 1.1  The internal market and integrated care:
summary of problems and solutions**

| Internal market | Integrated care |
|---|---|
| Fragmented responsibility; little strategic planning. | Jointly agreed HIPs. |
| Competition between hospitals; variations in who is treated. | Co-operation to replace competition; patients treated according to need. |
| Sharing best practice inhibited by ethos of competition; quality variable. | New mechanisms to share best practice; performance framework to improve quality. |
| Perverse incentives of efficiency index; budgets artificially partitioned. | Efficiency index replaced by reference costs; unified budgets. |
| High administrative costs. | Management costs capped; transaction costs cut. |
| Short-term contracts focussing cost and volume. | Longer-term service agreements linked to quality improvements. |
| NHS Trusts run as secretive businesses with unrepresentative boards; primary legal duty on finance. | NHS Trusts with representative boards, open meetings; new legal duties on quality. |

*Source:* Adapted from *The New NHS* (DoH, 1997a, section 2.24).

At home, improved information and advice will be available through a new 24-hour telephone helpline, NHS Direct. Pilots began in 1998 and the expectation is that the whole country will be covered by 2000. In the community, an improvement in advice and treatment will be facilitated by connecting GP surgeries to hospitals through NHSnet. Demonstration sites were established in 1998, with 2002 given as the date for national availability. In hospital, access to specialist services for those with suspected cancer will take two weeks from the time of referral by a GP.

This timeframe will apply to people with breast cancer from April 1999, and to people with all other forms of cancer by 2000.

In February 1998, the Green Paper *Our Healthier Nation* (DoH, 1998d) was published. It described the 'new public health', a framework for improving health and strengthening the public health role of the NHS. In this document, the causes of ill health are categorised under the headings 'fixed', 'social and economic', 'environmental', 'lifestyle', and 'access to services' (*ibid.,* section 2.3). The personal, social and economic arguments for improving health are outlined, and the notion of 'contracts for health' is introduced. In the proposed national contracts, the underlying principle is that everyone has a contribution to make towards achieving the policy goals. Also, the action that various stakeholders can take is suggested. The two key aims are:

- to improve the health of the population as a whole by increasing the length of people's lives and the number of years people spend free from illness; and,
- to improve the health of the worst off in society and to narrow the health gap (*ibid.,* section 3.10).

The document identifies four priority areas: heart disease and stroke, accidents, cancer, and mental health. Within each priority area, national targets are set and a national contract is described. It is stated that the main task of government in these national contracts is to tackle the root causes of ill health (social, economic and environmental) through the implementation of their overall policies. The fight against joblessness forms part of the overall strategy. Within this strategy, the Welfare to Work Budget is being used to fund the New Deal initiative for young people, the long-term unemployed and lone parents, along with its extension to people with disabilities and people with long-standing illness. Social exclusion is to be tackled through the work of the newly established Social Exclusion Unit and with the support of social services departments (see DoH, 1998e). Another initiative targeted on deprived areas is the establishment of a network of healthy living centres across the country, funded by money from the National Lottery Charities Board. These centres are intended to support the overall aims of the public health agenda, and to provide local communities with opportunities to become involved. Three settings offering opportunities to improve health and reduce health inequalities are identified:

- healthy schools – focusing on children;
- healthy workplaces – focusing on adults; and,
- healthy neighbourhoods – focusing on older people (DoH, 1998d, see section 3.71).

In relation to mental health, the Green Paper widened debate about risk factors to include the influence of social and environmental factors. The targets, however, were limited to reducing the death rate from suicide and undetermined injury amongst people with severe mental illness by 17% by the year 2010, with intermediate targets for 2005. This focus on suicide rate reduction builds on the earlier *Health of the Nation* (DoH, 1993a; 1994b) targets. The modesty of the public health targets is justified on the grounds that setting clear, achievable priorities is the best strategy to bring about real measurable improvements.

In July 1999, the subsequent public health White Paper *Saving Lives: Our Healthier Nation* (DoH, 1999c) was published. The four priority areas are maintained, along with the overall aims of the policy. This White Paper is described as an 'action plan for tackling poor health and improving the health of everyone in England, especially the worst off' (*ibid.*, para. 1.2). Progress towards these aims is to be assessed through the use of health impact assessments. The government's proposed 'third way' in public health is linked to the idea of achieving a new balance between individual action and wider action, involving partnership between individuals, communities and government (*ibid.*, para. 1.32).

In *Saving Lives* (DoH, 1999c), a summary is given of investment in the health and social care modernisation programme. In addition to the £21 billion made available for the health reforms through the Comprehensive Spending Review (DoH, 1998c), details are provided of investment linked to the goal of producing a healthier population:

- £110 million to help people give up smoking;
- £300 million to develop healthy living centres (from the National Lottery);
- £290 million for health action zones;
- £54 million to develop NHS Direct; and,
- £96 million through a Public Health Development Fund (to implement the public health White Paper) (DoH, 1999c, see para. 1.7).

This investment is to be used primarily to reduce health inequalities caused by poverty and social exclusion, and to focus on achieving the targets set for the four priority areas. Also, there is a commitment to raise standards;

reactivate the duty of the NHS to promote good health; establish a Health Development Agency; and, reduce smoking. To ensure that people have the information they need to make healthy decisions the government announced the Healthy Citizen's Programme. This initiative has three main strands: NHS Direct, health skills, and expert patients. The need to address issues relating to ethnicity is highlighted in connection with: the poor health experienced by people in some minority ethnic groups, including poor mental health; the lack of access to appropriate services; and, to racial discrimination.

The target to be achieved by the year 2010 with respect to mental illness is 'to reduce the death rate from suicide and undetermined injury by at least a fifth' (*ibid*, para. 1.5). The selection of this target is discussed in the White Paper in relation to the point raised in the consultation exercise, that a morbidity target would be better than a mortality target. However, it is argued that no solution was put forward to solve the problem of how to measure or monitor the suggested morbidity targets, and that there are benefits associated with the chosen mortality targets (*ibid,* chapter 8). The links between mental illness and risk factors for physical illness, including the priority areas of cancer and heart disease, are noted in *Saving Lives,* along with the estimated economic costs of mental ill health. To promote mental health and social inclusion, the government states that mental health must be one of the key outcomes of each of its major policies.

The social services White Paper *Modernising Social Services* (DoH, 1998e), set out the 'third way' for social services departments. In this document, the 'third way' is described as one that 'moves the focus away from who provides the care, and places it firmly on the quality of services experienced by, and outcomes achieved for, individuals and their carers and families (*ibid.,* section 1.7). This White Paper focuses on the need to:

- promote independence and social inclusion;
- improve protection; and,
- raise standards.

Added to these central concerns, are the priority areas identified in relation to services for adults, which include:

- improving consistency; and,
- providing convenient, user-centred services.

These policy goals are to be achieved through better regulation to protect vulnerable people; improved professional standards and training; working in partnership with other organisations, especially the NHS; and, the introduction of performance management arrangements. Performance management will use 'best value' principles, along with national performance standards and targets. Best value is the system introduced to replace compulsory competitive tendering. The intention is to secure the 'best suppliers' of services and, thereby, improve quality (DoH, 1999d, section 4.10). Commissions for Care Standards will be set up in each of the eight health regions to replace the existing system for inspection and regulation of care homes. A long-term care charter is to be developed, together with better information and a 'fair access to care' initiative. Local authority social services have been given a duty of partnership, and a duty to promote the economic and social well being of their areas. The duty of partnership will be facilitated by the abolition of the internal market; the proposed 'pooled budgets' for joint commissioning of services; and, the additional funds made available for partnership working. Health authorities have lead responsibility for consulting with NHS Trusts, PCGs, other primary care professionals, and the public. For local authority social services, a specific target has been set in relation to improving independence for service users through employment. Employment is described as an important pathway to independence and reducing social exclusion. This emphasis on promoting independence through employment is linked to the government's New Deal initiative and the proposed Single Gateway for disabled people (see also DoH, 1998d above). Other government initiatives such as the New Deal for Communities will underpin the work of social services departments in promoting independence and reducing social exclusion.

**Improving Quality**

The government has stated that: 'the new NHS will have quality at its heart' (DoH, 1997a, section 3.2). The framework for improving quality was outlined in the Consultation Paper *A First Class Service* (DoH, 1998f), which described how standards are to be 'set nationally, delivered locally and monitored externally'. This new focus on quality is intended to give patients the 'twin guarantee of consistency and responsiveness' (*ibid*, section 6.8). Quality is interpreted widely to refer to 'the quality of the patient's experience as well as the clinical result' (*ibid*, section 3.2). The government is committed to improve performance and raise standards throughout the NHS by improving quality and effectiveness, efficiency and pay (DoH, 1998c, section 7.7). Structurally, quality will be delivered at national and local levels, and through the establishment of a new organisation to deal with shortcomings in the system.

*National Service Frameworks and the National Institute of Clinical Excellence*

Nationally, national service frameworks (NSF) will be introduced to standardise consistency of access and quality of care, drawing on the best available evidence and the views of service users. Also, the National Institute of Clinical Excellence (NICE) will be set up to provide guidance on the clinical and cost-effectiveness of various drugs and therapies, and to disseminate this information throughout the NHS. Good practice will be highlighted through the beacon services initiative. Locally, PCGs comprised of local doctors and nurses, will plan and commission services in line with local population needs and national standards. Local service agreements will reflect these quality standards and national targets.

*Clinical Governance and the Commission for Health Improvement*

Clinical standards will be ensured through the introduction of a new clinical governance system to NHS Trusts and primary care. The Commission for Health Improvement (CHI) has been set up to oversee the delivery of quality in clinical services and to intervene where problems emerge. It is intended to complement the clinical governance system. Clinical governance is a new system introduced to guarantee that quality is at the core of the NHS. It is intended that clinical governance will build on the long-standing role of professionals and statutory bodies in setting, promoting and regulating standards. It is a way of making the NHS more accountable for the quality of services it provides and for maintaining standards. The concept of clinical governance incorporates elements of life-long learning, professional self-regulation, and external monitoring. Legislation is to be introduced to give NHS Trusts a new duty for quality of care. Chief Executives of NHS Trusts will be held accountable for ensuring that clinical governance systems are in place and are effectively implemented.

*Efficiency and Effectiveness*

The government's intention is that efficiency and effectiveness should be linked to quality improvement (*ibid.,* section 7.7). To this end, a new performance framework has been developed. The new National Performance Framework focuses on six key areas to measure performance:

- health improvement;
- fair access;
- effective delivery of appropriate healthcare;
- efficiency;
- patient and carer experience; and,
- health outcomes of NHS care (DoH, 1997a, see section 8.5).

New information technology will be introduced to support the desired quality and efficiency gains planned for the NHS. Accordingly this will mean that:

- patient records will be available electronically;
- NHSnet will speed up the process of obtaining information, and accessing treatment and care;
- accurate information about finance and performance will be available;
- knowledge about health, illness and best practice will be available on the Internet; and,
- telemedicine will be developed (*ibid.,* see section 3.15).

In summary, five ways in which efficient and effective use of resources will be safeguarded include:

- the introduction of a single, unified budget for health and community services, prescribing, and the development of primary care infrastructure that aligns financial and clinical responsibility in PCGs;
- in both health authorities and PCGs, management costs will be capped, and performance will be benchmarked;
- NHS Trusts will be required to publish costs for treatments they provide, and a schedule of costs across the country will be published to allow comparisons of efficiency;
- incentives to improve performance and efficiency will be provided in the form of cash benefits to NHS Trusts and PCGs. Savings made from longer-term agreements will be available to improve services; and,

- sanctions will be available in situations where performance fails to meet required standards - health authorities will be able to withdraw freedoms from PCGs; PCGS will be able to change providers if necessary; the NHS Executive will have the power to intervene to improve performance; and, the Secretary of State can remove the Trust Board (*ibid.*, see sections 3.8 - 3.13).

## *Health Action Zones*

Health Action Zones (HAZ) are initiatives designed to give priority to areas with the greatest needs and to target inequalities in health (DoH, 1998d, section 3.51). They are expected to have a duration of between five and ten years so that they can realise opportunities to develop new partnerships and to put plans into action. They are expected to 'bring together organisations within and beyond the NHS to develop and implement a locally agreed strategy for improving the health of local people' (DoH, 1997a, section 4.19). Initially, up to ten HAZ were set up from April 1998 to act as pilots.

## *Health Improvement Programmes*

Health Improvement Programmes (HIPs) are local strategies to deliver national targets for improving health and healthcare at local level. In addition, they have a role to play in reducing inequalities in health and focusing on those who experience social exclusion. HIPs are the plans for each locality to contribute to the national contracts for health (DoH, 1998d; 1999c). HIPS will cover:

- how the most important health needs of the local population will be met by the NHS and other partners through public health measures;
- how the main healthcare requirements will be met directly by NHS service provision or through joint provision with social services; and,
- the range, location and investment required for local health services to meet the identified needs (DoH, 1997a, see section 4.9).

HIPs will last for a period of three-years and will be updated as appropriate on the basis of annual reviews. HIPs will provide a framework within which PCGs will commission services for the local community. HIPs will include targets and standards for performance. These targets will be agreed between health authorities and PCGs, and progress will be monitored against them. The targets will be built into service agreements with NHS

Trusts, and will be used to hold Trusts to account for delivery against the HIP. Health authorities will have lead responsibility for drawing-up HIPs, in consultation with NHS Trusts, PCGs and other primary care professionals. Local NHS organisations have been given a statutory duty of partnership that extends to local authorities. Health authorities will monitor the implementation of the HIPs and will have reserve powers to ensure that major investments are in line with the agreed plan. Health authorities also have responsibilities for partnership working in relation to plans for education and training of the local workforce, and for co-ordinating the planned introduction of information technology.

## Primary Care Groups

PCGs bring together doctors, nurses and others in each area to plan and commission services for local populations. They are intended to develop around natural communities, yet take advantage of co-terminosity where appropriate. Typically, PCGs are expected to serve local populations of about 100,000 patients. Each PCG will have available to it their population's share of resources for health and community health services, prescribing and developing GP infrastructure.

The government has emphasised that PCGs grew out of a range of commissioning models, which included locality commissioning groups, GP fundholding and multifunds. PCGs will build on what was good within these models and locate those lessons within the framework provided by the HIPs. This will mean that the benefit of systems like fundholding can be shared amongst all patients without the associated disadvantages. The functions of PCGs can be briefly summarised:

- to use knowledge of local needs to contribute to the HIP;
- to work in partnership to promote the health of the local population;
- to commission health services for their local populations in line with the HIP;
- to monitor performance against service agreements;
- to develop primary care by joint working, including developing clinical governance; and,
- to better integrate primary and community health services and work more closely with social services (*ibid.,* see section 5.9).

As part of the implementation of clinical governance in the NHS, PCGs will be expected to nominate a senior professional to take lead responsibility for standards and professional development within the Group. This expectation will similarly extend to individual practices. The precise form PCGs adopt will depend on existing arrangements, and on the iterative learning process as they develop over time. Four options are available to PCGS:

- support the Health Authority in commissioning care;
- take devolved responsibility for managing the budget for healthcare;
- become freestanding bodies accountable to the health authority for commissioning care; or
- become freestanding bodies accountable to the health authority for commissioning care and for providing community health services locally (*ibid.,* see section 5.11).

The intention is that the new arrangements will result in PCGs developing prompt, accessible and responsive services for the local population. In addition, they will be encouraged to be active in community development and improving health in general. New legislation has been introduced to establish PCTs, for those PCGs capable of becoming freestanding (House of Commons, 1999). NHS Trusts and PCTs may combine if appropriate. However, the new PCTs are not expected to be responsible for mental health or learning disability services, although they will be responsible for commissioning these services. The reason given for this is that, in the case of mental health, health and social care boundaries are not fixed, joint working is extremely important, and an integrated range of provision is needed. Specialist mental health and learning disability Trusts are considered to be the best way to co-ordinate service delivery.

*The Role of Health Authorities*

In the planned reform of the NHS, health authorities will be given a strategic leadership role. Their main objectives will be to improve overall health and to reduce inequalities. Health authorities will retain their public health responsibilities. In addition, they will incorporate the 'public health approach', outlined in *Our Healthier Nation* (DoH, 1998d) and *Saving Lives* (DoH, 1999c), with targets in four priority areas. The report of the Director of Public Health will be used in the development of the HIP. As mentioned above, health authorities will be required to work in partnership with local authorities and others, through a new statutory duty of partnership. They will be expected to plan with others to secure local action to improve health in relation to social, environmental and economic issues. The key tasks associated with the functions of health authorities are to:

- assess the health needs of the local population;
- link this assessment to the strategy outlined in the HIP and developed in partnership;
- decide on the range and location of local healthcare services in line with the HIP;
- set local targets and standards for quality and efficiency in the context of national guidance;
- support the development of PCGs;
- allocate resources to PCGs; and,
- hold PGCs to account for their performance (DOH, 1997a, see section 4.3).

Health authorities will co-operate with local social services to plan patient care, especially for people with continuing health and social care needs, in order to provide integrated continuing and community care services. Plans for pooling budgets in relation to people with disabilities or mental health problems are being explored because it is recognised that their needs span health and social care services.

To rebuild public confidence, health authorities have an important role in consulting with local people and involving them in decision-making. In addition, it is envisaged that HAZ will offer 'opportunities to explore new ways of involving local people'. Health authorities will:

- involve the public in developing the HIP;
- ensure that PCGs have effective arrangements for public involvement; and,
- publish agreed strategies, targets and details of progress against them (*ibid.*, see section 4.19).

## The Mental Health Reforms

For over forty years, the aim of mental health policy has been to shift the balance of service provision and accommodation for people with mental illness away from institutions and towards the community. Within that time, a repeated observation has been that progress in translating community care policy goals into practice has been slow and patchy across the country. Plans to close the old psychiatric hospitals resulted in the resettlement of many long-stay patients in the community, but ran into problems achieving the ultimate goal of closure, with many still remaining open and facing rising unit costs. In these instances, transferring funds for the development of community services was thwarted, although subsequent initiatives such as the Mental Illness Specific Grant (Caring for People, 1989) were introduced in an attempt to ameliorate this situation. More recently, despite renewed enthusiasm for care in the community with the introduction of the *NHS and Community Care Act* (House of Commons, 1990), tragedies involving people with serious mental illness have received extensive, negative media coverage. In response, the government of the day announced their plans for more coercive measures to manage risk in the community (e.g. DoH, 1994a; House of Commons, 1996). New Labour's assessment of the situation is clearly stated in the mental health White Paper:

> Care in the community has failed because, while it improved the treatment of many people who were mentally ill, it left far too many walking the streets, often at risk to themselves and a nuisance to others. A small but significant minority have been a threat to others or themselves (DoH, 1998b, Foreword).

The opening chapter to *Modernising Mental Health Services* (DoH, 1998b) begins by discussing three themes:

- the importance of good mental health;
- stigma of mental illness; and,
- the need for modernisation of mental health services.

Then, the fear of mental illness, the extent of mental ill health in the population, and the risk factors associated with mental illness, are briefly reviewed. Consistent with the public health orientation of the health and social care reforms, the social, environmental, economic and biological factors linked to causation in mental illness, are acknowledged. Attention then focuses on mental illness and suicide, and mental illness and homicide. The suicide rate is reported to be falling, but there are still over 4,000 deaths per year in England. It is pointed out that this masks variation between different groups of people in the population. Groups at higher risk of committing suicide include: young men, people with a history of self-harm and severe mental illness, unemployed people, people who have suffered loss or bereavement, people detained in prison, various occupational groups, and young women from the Indian sub-continent. Figures given for homicides in England and Wales are taken from 1994, with 476 convictions cited, of which 61 are attributed to people with mental illness. Information from the National Confidential Inquiry (Appleby, 1997) is used to show the links between factors such as contact with specialist services, co-morbidity, compliance and so on (see Table 1.2). More recent research has since been published (Appleby *et al.*, 1999; Shaw *et al.*, 1999).

**Table 1.2  Mental illness and suicide and mental illness and homicide**

|  | Mental illness and suicide | Mental illness and homicide |
|---|---|---|
| **Contact with services** | 26% in contact in previous year | 12%* in contact at the time |
| **Co-morbidity** | 50% with another problem – substance misuse, personality disorder, or combination | 26%* with another problem drug or alcohol misuse, personality disorder, or combination |
| **Discharged from Hospital** | 28% discharged in previous three months | |
| **Compliant with Treatment** | < 50% | |

**\*Based on cumulative figures relating to several years**
*Source:* Adapted from *Modernising Mental Health Services* (DoH, 1998b, section 1.8 – 1.9).

Despite the large number of suicides each year in comparison to the numbers of people with mental illness who commit homicide, the government states that:

> Whilst adverse media reporting can distort the relationship between mental illness and homicide, the public have a right to be concerned (*ibid.*, section 1.10).

*Modernising Mental Health Services* (DoH, 1998b, p.32) lists three key themes associated with modernising mental health and social care:

- improving services;
- improving safety; and,
- involving patients, users and carers.

The vision for modern mental health services is built on the wider health and social care policy developments, with the promotion of partnership working to produce integrated care.

**Table 1.3  The health and social care modernisation agenda**

| Modernising health services | Modernising social services |
| --- | --- |
| Tackle the root causes of ill health. | Promote people's independence. |
| Raise standards to provide a high quality of excellent health care. | Raise standards across the whole of social care everywhere. |
| Provide treatment and care quickly and more conveniently | Improve protection of vulnerable people |

Partnership working is central to integrated health and social care

*Source:* DoH (1998c, section 2.2).

Overlap between the health and social care policies and mental health policy is specifically related to improving the quality and consistency of service provision; reducing inequalities in health, and in access to health care; developing links with housing and rehabilitation services; and, encouraging employment amongst service users. The government's proposals for modernising mental health services involve three interlocking elements: investment, the national service framework, and legislative reform. *Modernising Mental Health Services* (DoH, 1998b) describes how quality and efficiency will be improved by targeting investment of £700 million where it is needed over a period of three years. Investment will be used to develop a comprehensive range of service provision across the country; monitor performance through a variety of structures and systems; and, set standards within the NSF (DoH, 1999a) for the care and treatment of mental illness. In addition, reform to the mental health legislative framework is underway (DoH, 1999b) to close perceived gaps in the system which limit the ability of professionals to effectively manage risk in the community. In particular, these risks are linked to a minority of individuals who are likely to refuse medication for their mental disorder, or who are deemed to have an 'untreatable' personality disorder. Also, the CPA system for supporting people with mental illness in the community has been revised (DoH, 1999f).

A key mechanism through which the government intends to achieve its aims is the introduction of the NSF (DoH, 1999a) for adults of working age with mental health problems (see below). This will provide the structure for the delivery of 'safe, sound and supportive' mental health services. Table 1.4 outlines the key elements within each of these dimensions.

*Safe Services*

In *Modernising Mental Health Services* (DoH, 1998b), safe services are described in terms of the need for good, timely assessments to effectively manage risk, and to provide early interventions and avoid crises. Reference is made to primary care and the need for education and training. The need to ensure that sufficient beds are available applies to the range of provision including 24-hour staffed beds, acute beds and secure beds. It is acknowledged that difficulties can be experienced in relation to all types of beds, with availability failing to meet demand and causing inappropriate placement. Local authority provision of residential, respite and day care is mentioned as an area to be developed with additional funding made available through the Mental Health Grant. Local authorities and the NHS are urged to work together to ensure the right mix of provision. Safety in hospital is mentioned, along with the need to reduce the number of mixed sex wards.

Better outreach, especially assertive outreach, is described as an effective treatment for avoiding unnecessary hospitalisation. Assertive outreach is identified as an essential component of safe care and treatment, and investment is to be targeted to expand this approach.

**Table 1.4  Key elements of safe, sound and supportive mental health services**

| Safe | Sound | Supportive |
|---|---|---|
| Good risk management. | 24-hour access. | Involvement of patients. |
| Early intervention. | Needs assessment. | Access to employment, education and housing. |
| Enough beds. | Good primary care. | Working in partnership. |
| Better outreach. | Effective treatment. | Better information. |
| Integrated forensic and secure provision. | Effective care processes. | Promoting good mental health and reducing stigma. |
| Modern legislative Framework. | | |

Source: Adapted from Modernising Mental Health Services (DoH, 1998b, chapter 4).

Plans to integrate forensic and secure provision are intended to improve the availability of secure provision, stem inappropriate placement, and deliver continuity of care. To this end, part of the Modernisation Funds are to be used to set up new commissioning teams in each region. Legislation will be passed to transform the existing Special Hospitals into NHS Trusts. Reform of the 1983 *Mental Health Act* (House of Commons, 1983) is underway (DoH, 1999b). The Act has been described as outdated and inappropriate for the pattern of contemporary service provision that is community-based. Further, important mention has been made of the need to review the responsibilities of patients to comply with their care and treatment regimes, and the future of the Mental Health Act Commission will be considered in the light of the role of the CHI. However, relevant work to date such as the Green Paper *Who Decides* (DoH, 1997b), and the subsequent White Paper *Making Decisions* (DoH, 1999e), will be taken into account in the process of reforming mental health legislation (DoH, 1999b).

In relation to people with severe personality disorder, a new form of reviewable detention is being considered in order to reduce the risk to the public posed by some people whose condition is outside the scope of the *Mental Health Act* (House of Commons, 1983). The principles that are informing this proposal are:

- the safety of the public is of prime concern;
- admission to the new regime will neither be dependent upon the person having committed an offence, nor whether they are treatable under the *Mental Health Act*;
- release into the community will depend upon a rigorous assessment that the person no longer poses a grave risk to the public;
- the regime will comply with the Government's obligations under the European Court of Human Rights (DoH, 1998b, see section 4.33).

The Green Paper *Reform of the Mental Health Act* (DoH, 1999b) presents further details of the proposals for consultation.

*Sound Services*

One of the key aims in the vision for modern mental health services is twenty-four hour access throughout the year. Accordingly, additional funding will be made available to develop this type of access. NHS Direct will play an important role in this strategy. In future, it is hoped that variation across the country will be due to variation in the assessed needs of local population. Shared population needs assessment is to form the basis for the development of the HIP, which will set out the plan for the commissioning of local services. Partners to the plan will develop a performance framework to monitor the achievement of their objectives. Individual needs assessment will follow on from this initial planning phase.

The important role of primary care in the treatment and management of mental illness is highlighted in relation to the development of PCG/Ts, and their responsibilities for working in partnership to plan, commission and deliver mental health services. These activities are to take place within the agreed framework of the HIP and the NSF, with specialist mental health services being commissioned from specialist providers. Clinical governance and clinical audit are the mechanisms for improving and maintaining quality in primary care.

Delivering effective treatment is viewed as essential to the provision of sound services. It is recognised that there is a need for information, education and training to achieve this goal. The NICE has been established to provide information to professionals about effective and cost-effective drugs and therapies, along with clinical guidelines and appropriate methodologies. Additional resources will be made available for the introduction of new drugs for schizophrenia. These resources will initially be targeted on those health authorities with the highest levels of mental illness in their populations. GPs will be supported in their prescribing by another government initiative, *PRODIGY*. This software aids decision-making in prescribing. The new unified budgets of PCGs are intended to act as an incentive to deliver 'the optimum package of care for each patient' (DoH, 1998b, section 4.44). The evidence base for various psychological therapies is discussed, and the point is made that these need to be targeted on those people likely to benefit. Particular mention is made of structured therapies in relation to depression and anxiety; and, cognitive behavioural techniques and family interventions, in relation to the management of delusions and hallucinations, and schizophrenia, respectively.

In terms of effective care processes, the care programme approach and the care management approach were intended to play a central role in the delivery of effective care and treatment. Although the difficulties experienced in practice are not explicitly referred to, they are implicit in the government's plan to review them. The findings from a study commissioned by the Department of Health are intended to cast light on how best to integrate these systems to deliver continuity of care, and some indication as to the relative cost-effectiveness of different models for achieving this goal. In reviewing these two approaches, the aim is to achieve consistency, proper focus on need, harmonise the two approaches and, importantly for targeting, streamline the process whereby the most vulnerable receive the care of the most expert.

*Supportive Services*

*Modernising Mental Health Services* (DoH, 1998b) states that good quality, supportive services are those that actively inform and involve patients, service users and carers in the processes of care and treatment. Good quality, 'therapeutic' relationships between patients and professionals are identified as the basis for effective interventions. It is noted that people with mental health problems should be treated according to need, and that they should have their autonomy and ability to make decisions respected, wherever possible. It is claimed that this will go some way to reduce the extent to which certain groups experience social exclusion, e.g. people from black and ethnic minority communities. Recognising the contribution made by carers, the government highlights the importance of involving them in joint decision-making with staff, patients and service users concerning care and treatment options. Also, comment is made that carers should be recognised as partners with local health and social care providers.

As part of their recovery, many people with mental health problems may need help to access work and education, or to find appropriate housing. Health authorities and social services departments are, therefore, urged to work closely with local housing authorities to address the housing needs of people with mental illness. In relation to accessing employment, it is stated that: 'for many people with a mental disorder, the best outcome will be to obtain and sustain meaningful work' (*ibid.*, section 4.53). To facilitate this and to remove existing barriers to participation in employment, the Employment Service, the Benefits Agency and others are being brought together, and the following initiatives have been introduced for people with disability:

- improved incentives on longer-term incapacity benefits will help them take a job;
- the Disabled Person's Tax Credit will help those whose earnings are limited by a long-term illness or disability; and,
- the new personal advisor scheme will greatly assist those who have difficulty coping with the employment system (*ibid.*, section 4.54).

Working in partnership is seen as essential for the delivery of effective NHS and social care in mental health services, because people with mental illness need the support of a range of services at various times. Their needs are not restricted to one type of service. HIPs are the intended means for making a reality of partnership working between professionals in primary care, specialist services, local authority services and other agencies. It is pointed out that social services staff currently work in partnership through their membership of multi-disciplinary teams such as community mental health teams, crisis teams, assertive outreach teams, and so on. They also work in partnership in their capacity as Approved Social Workers, providers of social care, and managers of community care budgets for mental health services. The government will make funds available to target social work training. In addition, partnerships between statutory and voluntary sector services (including charities) are encouraged. It is acknowledged that the voluntary sector has a lot to contribute in terms of its track record of successfully providing services, often to groups of people that statutory services find difficult to engage.

The importance of better information and improved communication for the provision of integrated mental health services is recognised, along with the opportunities this creates for partnership working at the interface between primary care and secondary specialist mental health services. Various initiatives will contribute to the availability of better information. These include the strategy for the NHS outlined in *Information for Health* (DoH/NHSE, 1998). This document sets targets for the implementation of electronic records in NHS Trusts and plans for the introduction of GP access to the NHS Net by 2002. These developments will improve the decision-making ability and risk management strategies of mental health professionals. Plans to integrate the care programme and care management systems are expected to help. The potential to include service utilisation data relating to mental health and social care in the Minimum Data Set, to aid service planning and delivery, is mentioned.

To combat the discrimination that people with mental health problems often experience in their day-to-day lives, the Department of Health is working with other organisations like the Health Education Authority to educate the public and reduce discrimination. Promoting mental health is also described as the business of employers, teachers and members of PCGs. Reducing stress at work and at school are important goals that are consistent with the overall public health approach outlined earlier (DoH, 1998d; 1999c). It is argued that PCGs are strategically well-placed to promote mental health through: raising awareness of mental health issues; developing initiatives to provide support to people in need or in crisis; and, arranging early referral to specialist secondary services when necessary. Standard 1 of the *National Service Framework for Mental Health* (DoH,

1999a) focuses on mental health promotion, which incorporates combating discrimination and promoting social inclusion. Unemployment and ethnicity are mentioned amongst the risk factors included in the rationale for this national standard. Suggested service models for individuals at risk of developing mental health problems, like the unemployed, include promoting the use of local self-help groups, and for vulnerable groups such as people from black and minority ethnic communities, the development of specific programmes. The work of the Social Exclusion Unit is a key initiative designed to promote mental health and reduce discrimination. A first priority for the Unit is to reduce the numbers of people sleeping rough. Another initiative expected to make a contribution to this goal is Sure Start, aimed at helping children from disadvantaged areas.

**National Service Framework**

The *National Service Framework for Mental Health* (DoH, 1999a) sets out the national standards for mental health services, and provides national service models to promote mental health and treat mental illness. In addition, it sets national milestones and identifies specific performance indicators by which the mental health reforms will be monitored. The NSF is intended to guide investment, and to provide information about the programmes that will underpin the work of local health and social care agencies. The introduction of the NSF is described as part of the drive to improve quality and reduce unacceptable variations. It refers to the 'mental health needs of working age adults up to 65' (*ibid.*, p.3). Implementation of the NSF will be funded by the extra £700 million to be made available over three years to reshape mental health services. In most areas, the first priority will be to continue to 'address the gaps in current services for people with severe and enduring mental illness', including access to 24-hour staffed accommodation and assertive outreach. In other areas, the focus will be on providing cost-effective services for people with common mental health problems (*ibid.*, p.4). The NSF outlines what people with mental health problems can expect from services:

- involve service users and their carers in planning and delivery of care;
- deliver high quality treatment and care which is known to be effective and appropriate;
- be well suited to those who use them and non-discriminatory;
- be accessible so that help can be obtained when and where it is needed;

- promote their safety and that of their carers, staff and the wider public;
- offer choices which promote independence;
- be well co-ordinated between all staff and agencies;
- deliver continuity of care for as long as this is needed;
- empower and support their staff; and,
- be properly accountable to the public, service users and carers (*ibid.*, Executive Summary).

The NSF sets seven national standards in five key areas, provides examples of service models and good practice, and indicates how performance against these standards will be assessed. The standards refer to:

Standard 1                    mental health promotion;

Standards 2 and 3        primary care and access to services;

Standards 4 and 5        effective services for people with severe mental illness;

Standard 6                    caring about carers; and,

Standard 7                    preventing suicide (DoH, 1999a, p.5).

National milestones outlined in the NSF refer to:

- HIPs demonstrating links between NHS organisations and other partners to promote mental health and combat discrimination and social exclusion;
- the production of clinical governance reports;
- the development of agreed protocols between primary care and specialist services for the management and treatment of a range of mental disorders;
- monitoring and review of prescribing of anti-depressants, anti-psychotics and benzodiazepines;
- integrated care plans with a responsible co-ordinator for people with severe mental illness;
- for people on enhanced CPA, the production of written care plans with details of how service users, carers and GPs can contact specialist mental health services around the clock;
- assertive outreach services for those on enhanced CPA or at risk of losing contact with services;
- a planned increase in secure beds;
- an increase in the percentage of community mental health teams, integrating health and social services staff within a single structure;
- local workforce strategies that ensure a review and action plan, an education and training plan, and a retention strategy; and,

- local information strategies that ensure: an action plan to implement information systems relating to people on the CPA, including access on a 'need to know' basis; implementation of the Mental Health Minimum Data Set by March 2003; and, an annual review of the appropriateness of bed use, with recommendations that are implemented (DoH, 1999a, Executive Summary).

Local milestones are intended to complement these national milestones. In addition to the targets set in relation to reducing the suicide rate, the NSF outlines other commitments of the government relevant to the mental health reforms. These include the reduction of the rate of psychiatric emergency admissions by 2% by April 2002; making NHS Direct available across the country by the end of 2002; and, eliminating mixed sex wards in 95% of health authorities by 2002.

## Targeting People with Severe and Enduring Mental Illness (SEMI)

Targeting people with SEMI for specialist intervention is an important theme underpinning the twin policy goals of improving 'safety' and 'quality' in the provision of mental health services. Targeting is not a new strategy. It can be traced to the 1983 *Mental Health Act* (House of Commons, 1983), Section 117 of which provided for the aftercare of people with mental illness discharged from hospital. Targeting has long been discussed in relation to the caseloads of community psychiatric nurses (Wooff *et al.*, 1986; White, 1990) and community mental health teams (Patmore and Weaver, 1991). Many CPNs and CMHTs have been found to be working with a significant proportion of people with less severe mental illness, and in some cases, to have no-one on their caseloads with a psychotic illness (Corney, 1999).

In the last decade, several initiatives were introduced that were designed to target resources on people with SEMI, in order to effectively manage risk in the community. The care programme approach (CPA), introduced in 1991, was intended to provide a framework for the care of people with mental illness discharged from hospital (DoH, 1990). Under the CPA, all people accepted for treatment by mental health services should be allocated a key worker who takes responsibility for assessing their health and social care needs, developing a care plan, involving all concerned in that plan, and reviewing the plan. In the following year, the *Health of the Nation* (DoH, 1993a) identified mental illness as a priority area, with goals to improve the health and social functioning of people with serious mental illness, and to reduce the suicide rate amongst them by the turn of the century.

However, in the wake of a series of incidents involving people with SEMI, the Department of Health reviewed its legal powers (DoH, 1993b). The conclusions of this review formed the basis for the *Ten Point Plan* (DoH, 1993c). This plan was designed to improve risk management in the community, and to ensure that people with SEMI would not fall through the 'net of care'. The cornerstones of the plan involved the introduction of Supervision Registers (DoH, 1994a) and the power of supervised discharge (House of Commons, 1996), both of which were intended to be situated within the context of the CPA (DoH, 1990). These legalistic measures were meant to complement the existing mental health law, including Guardianship, and were supplemented with new guidance on discharge (DoH, 1994c).

However, in 1994, the Audit Commission published its review of mental health services in which it reported that 'resources are not well allocated, nor spent on the right mix of services and not targeted on the right people' (Audit Commission, 1994, p.54). The report stated that Department of Health policy was that:

> ...specialist psychiatric services should target their efforts on severely mentally ill people and ensure that they receive the treatment, care and follow-up they need and do not drift out of contact with services' (*ibid.*, p.5).

People with 'less severe' mental illness, the Report argued, should be cared for by primary care, who would need to be adequately supported in this task.

Several of the policy initiatives of the 1990s have been criticised in terms of the ethics, legality and likely effectiveness of the proposed measures. Although the CPA was expected to ensure that the health and social care needs of people with SEMI were assessed and met, this system was only slowly and inadequately implemented across the country (Mental Health Task Force, 1994). Also, the proposed integration of the CPA and care management approach has long awaited implementation in most areas (Audit Commission, 1994; Mental Health Act Commission, 1997). Various authors questioned whether initiatives like Supervision Registers are primarily about care or control, and pointed out that these registers are no substitute for adequate resources and services (Coffey, 1995; Eastman, 1994; Harrison, 1994; Kingdon, 1996). Others have highlighted the ambiguities inherent in the criteria for inclusion on Supervision Registers (Caldicott, 1994; Harrison and Bartlett, 1994), together with the anti-therapeutic nature of both Supervised Discharge Orders (Eastman, 1995) and Supervision Registers (Coffey, 1995).

The mental health modernisation programme continues the trend in national policy to target people with SEMI for specialist intervention, with people with 'less severe' mental illness being cared for in primary care. Additional investment is available to implement the policy, and legislative reform is on the way. In the NSF, Standards 4 and 5 focus on people with SEMI. These national standards identify what people with SEMI can expect from mental health services:

- receive care which optimises engagement, anticipates or prevents a crisis, and reduces risk;
- have a copy of a written care plan which: includes the action to be taken in a crisis by the service user, their carer, and their care co-ordinator;
- advise the GP how they should respond if the service user needs additional help and is regularly reviewed by their care co-ordinator; and,
- be able to access services 24 hours a day, 365 days a year (DoH, 1999a, Standard 4).

Standard 5 states that people assessed as requiring treatment away from home should have:

- timely access to an appropriate hospital bed or alternative bed or place, which is: in the least restrictive environment consistent with the need to protect them and the public; and, as close to home as possible; and,
- a copy of a written after care plan agreed on discharge, which sets out the care and rehabilitation to be provided, identifies the care co-ordinator, and specifies the action to be taken in a crisis (DoH, 1999a, p.51).

The government's proposals for a new *Mental Health Act* in which the safety of individuals and the public are of prime concern are outlined in the Green Paper *Reform of the Mental Health Act* (DoH, 1999b). In addition, the CPA has been revised with the intention of simplifying and clarifying the process whereby mentally ill people are supported in the community, and laying emphasis on the provision of a seamless service in which health and social care are integrated. In future, there will be two levels of CPA, standard and enhanced (DoH, 1999f).

## Conclusion

The policy context for mental health services as we enter the 21$^{ST}$ century is based on the belief that community care has failed, and that what is needed is root and branch reform to improve quality, but most especially, to ensure public safety. The health and social care reforms aim to put the 'national' back in the NHS, to raise standards, improve quality, and make a reality of joint-working in a primary care-led NHS. Although the modernisation of mental health services is integrated into these reforms, what is different in mental health policy is that the safety agenda is an important driving force behind the way services are to be planned, commissioned and delivered. Improving safety is linked to various initiatives described above. These include:

- the additional investment for the development of comprehensive mental health services, and for training and education in primary care;
- the introduction of the NSF;
- the encouragement for partnership working;
- the work of NICE in relation to effective drugs and therapies;
- the improvement of secure services; and
- the reform of mental health legislation.

Modernising mental health and improving safety is also linked to the directive to target specialist resources on people with SEMI. This strategy is built upon concern about how best to effectively manage risk in the community. During a decade of perceived breakdowns in care in the 1990s, as people 'slipped through the net' with apparent regularity, mental health policy introduced greater elements of social control. New Labour's policy agenda will continue that trend, with the introduction of more assertive and custodial forms of services and provision, together with the reform of mental health legislation.

However, whilst targeting people with SEMI for specialist intervention may be a rational strategy, many questions remain about how this will be achieved, and the potential contradiction that exists between this approach and other goals of mental health policy and practice. For example, how does greater coercion in mental health care affect the dynamics of the therapeutic relationship between practitioners and patients? How does targeting people with SEMI affect the policy goal to reduce stigma and discrimination? How is the SEMI population to be accurately defined and 'targeted', and by whom? Although structures and systems are being established to provide guidance in the care and treatment of mental illness, models of service delivery and so on, what models of collaboration will be advocated for the all important primary care/ specialist mental health services interface? Also, if mental health policy is to be 'outcome driven', what are the outcomes, and from whose perspective are they to be judged? Despite the investment of substantial resources in the development of the *Health of the Nation Outcome Scales* (Wing *et al.*, 1998), recent papers in the *British Medical Journal* (see e.g. Bebbington *et al.*, 1999; Sharma *et al.*, 1999) highlight numerous difficulties with this instrument.

Another issue concerns the contradiction between the explicit reference to the need to combat the stigmatisation and discrimination experienced by people with mental illness (DoH, 1998b; 1999a), and the reinforcement of negative stereotypes of serious mental illness by the government. This is evident in the way that the statistics about homicide and mental illness are presented and analysed. In contrast to the statistics for suicide in England, the numbers of people with mental illness who commit acts of homicide are small, even when they relate to England *and* Wales, *and* are based on cumulative figures from 1994 onwards. Further, these figures are presented in isolation from the evidence that the trend in homicides committed by mentally ill people is declining (Taylor and Gunn, 1999). Nevertheless, the government asserts that the public are 'right to be concerned' (DoH, 1998b, section 1.10). In formulating policy and seeking to educate the public, the government would be seen to act consistently were it to adopt the evidence-based approach they advocate for those responsible for policy implementation. As Taylor and Gunn (1999) cogently argue, mental health policy is currently driven by a misperception of the facts about homicide and people with serious mental illness. The Audit Commission report of 1994 was clear about this point:

> A popular perception is that community care is not working and that it is a cause both of danger to the public and of more mentally ill people on the streets... although the few [people with mental illness] who are dangerous need special attention in order to avoid any further tragedies, most people with schizophrenia lead relatively normal lives. Many are quiet and withdrawn and find it hard to cope with the demands of everyday life... In the last two decades of the community care policy the number of homicides committed by mentally ill people has not increased while the number committed by others has more than doubled (Audit Commission, 1994, section 10-13).

Others have commented on the tendency of the modernisation agenda to focus on the 'pursuit of the unobtainable': total safety in community care. Clearly, no form of provision is foolproof and at least this government is providing much needed resources and direction to implement its policy goals. For that they should be praised. Nevertheless, it remains problematic that worthy goals are justified by blanket statements concerning the failure of community care, and misrepresentation of the facts about the supposed dangers posed by people with mental illness based on an uncritical acceptance of the prejudices of the media.

The policy documents make clear that the majority of people with mental illness, people with 'less severe' mental illness, are to be cared for in primary care. Whilst this is in line with much health and social care provision, and is likely to be potentially less stigmatising, various problems remain. The term 'less severe' can be misleading. Many people so described have been found to have considerable, often long-term, problems (Bowers, 1997). Some of the money to be invested in mental health is to be ear-marked to improve the training of GPs and other primary care staff, and partnership working with other agencies is a requirement (DoH, 1997a; 1998b). This appears to make good sense, given the poor track record of GPs in accurately recognising and treating mental illness, working in multi-disciplinary teams, and joint-working with other sectors of care (see e.g. Audit Commission, 1994; West and Field, 1995).

From this brief concluding discussion, it would seem that, although there is much to applaud in the government's proposals for reform, there may be unintended consequences resulting from the 'public safety' orientation of its plans for mental health policy and practice. Nevertheless, amongst other positive changes, there is long-overdue investment in mental health, to translate policy goals into action; a national framework for improving quality and effectiveness; and, guidance in treatment decisions and service configurations. The strategy of targeting people with SEMI remains an important feature of mental health policy and practice. The multi-faceted, multi-disciplinary nature of this endeavour is reflected in the contributed chapters of this book, which bring together theory, policy and practice from different perspectives and disciplines within mental health.

## Acknowledgements

Crown copyright material is reproduced with the permission of the Controller of Her Majesty's Stationery Office.
Material from the Audit Commission Report *Finding a Place* (1994) is reproduced with kind permission of the Audit Commission.

# References

Appleby, L. (1997), *National Confidential Inquiry into Suicide and Homicide by People with Mental Illness: Progress Report,* Department of Health, London.
Appleby, L., Shaw, J., Amos, T., McDonnell, R., Harris, C., McKann, K., Kiernan, K., Davies, S., Bickley, H. and Parsons, R. (1999), 'Suicide Within 12 Months of Contact with Mental Health Services: National Clinical Survey', *British Medical Journal,* vol. 318, no. 18, pp. 1235-9.
Audit Commission (1994), *Finding a Place: A Review of Mental Health Services for Adults,* Audit Commission, London.
Bebbington, P., Bruga, T., Hill, T., Marsden, L, and Window, S. (1999), 'Validation of the Health of the Nation Outcome Scales', *British Journal of Psychiatry,* vol. 174, pp. 389-94.
Bowers, L. (1997), 'Community Psychiatric Nurse Caseloads and the 'Worried Well': Misspent Time or Vital Work?', *Journal of Advanced Nursing,* 26, pp. 930-6.
Caldicott, F. (1994), 'Supervision Registers: The College's Response', *Psychiatric Bulletin,* 18, pp. 383-8.
Caring for People (1989), *Caring for People: The Next Decade and Beyond,* Department of Health, London.
Coffey, M. (1995), 'Supervision Registers and Mental Health Problems', *Nursing Times,* 12 July, 91, (28), pp. 36-7.
Corney, R, (1999), 'Mental Health Services in Primary Care: The Overlap in Professional Roles', *Journal of Mental Health,* vol. 8, no. 2, pp. 187-94.
Department of Health (1990), Joint Health and Social Services Circular *Health and Social Services Development: "Caring for People" The Care Programme Approach for People with a Mental Illness referred to the Special Psychiatric Services* HC(90)23/LASSL(90)11, Department of Health, London.
Department of Health (1993a), *Health of the Nation Key Area Handbook Mental Illness,* Department of Health, London.
Department of Health (1993b), *Legal Powers on the Care of Mentally Ill People in the Community,* Department of Health, London.
Department of Health (1993c), 'Legislation Planned to Provide Supervised Discharge of Psychiatric Patients', *Press Release* (H93/908), HMSO, London.
Department of Health (1994a), *Introduction of Supervision Registers for Mentally Ill People from 1 April 1994 (HSG(94)5),* Department of Health, Fleetwood.
Department of Health (1994b), *Health of the Nation Key Area Handbook Mental Illness Second Edition,* Department of Health, London.
Department of Health (1994c), *Guidance on the Discharge from Hospital of Mentally Disordered People and Their Continuing Care in the Community,* Department of Health, Fleetwood.
Department of Health (1997a), *The New NHS: Modern, Dependable,* The Stationery Office (Cm. 3807), London.

Department of Health (1997b), *Who Decides? Making Decisions on Behalf of Mentally Incapacitated Adults,* HMSO, London.

Department of Health (1998a), 'Modernising Health and Social Services: National Priorities Guidance 1999/00 – 2001/02', *Health Service Circular Local Authority Circular, HSC 1998/159,* Department of Health, London.

Department of Health (1998b), *Modernising Mental Health Services, Safe, Sound and Supportive,* Department of Health, London.

Department of Health (1998c), *Modern Public Services for Britain: Investing in Reform,* The Stationery Office (Cm 4011), London.

Department of Health (1998d), *Our Healthier Nation: A Contract for Health,* The Stationery Office (Cm. 3852), London.

Department of Health (1998e), *Modernising Social Services,* The Stationery Office (Cm 4169), London.

Department of Health (1998f), *A First Class Service,* Department of Health, London.

Department of Health (1999a), *National Service Framework for Mental Health,* Department of Health, London.

Department of Health (1999b), *Reform of the Mental Health Act 1983 Proposals for Consultation,* The Stationery Office (Cm. 4480), London.

Department of Health (1999c), *Saving Lives: Our Healthier Nation,* The Stationery Office (Cm 4386), London.

Department of Health (1999d), *Modernising Government,* The Stationery Office (Cm 4310), London.

Department of Health (1999e), *Making Decisions,* Department of Health, London.

Department of Health (1999f), *Effective Care Co-ordination in Mental Health Services: A Policy Booklet,* SSI/NHSE, Department of Health, London.

Department of Health/ NHSE (1998), *Information for Health: An Information Strategy for the Modern NHS 1998-2005 A National Strategy for Local Implementation,* Department of Health, London.

Eastman, N. (1994), 'Mental Health Law: Civil Liberties and the Principle of Reciprocity', *British Medical Journal,* 1ST January, vol. 308, pp. 43-5.

Eastman, N. (1995), 'Anti-therapeutic Community Mental Health Law', *British Medical Journal,* 29th April, vol. 310, pp. 1081-2.

Gask, L., Sibbald, B. and Creed, F. (1997), 'Evaluating Models of Working at the Interface Between Mental Health Services and Primary Care', *British Journal of Psychiatry,* vol. 170, pp. 6-11.

Harrison, G. (1994), 'Supervision Registers: Unethical, Illegal and Unenforceable', *Mental Health Nursing,* 14, (5), pp. 6-8.

Harrison, G. and Bartlett, P. (1994), 'Supervision Registers for Mentally Ill People', *British Medical Journal,* vol. 309, pp. 551-2.

House of Commons (1983), *The Mental Health Act,* HMSO, London.

House of Commons (1990), *The NHS and Community Care Act,* HMSO, London.

House of Commons (1996), *Mental Health (Patients in the Community) Act,* HMSO, London.

House of Commons (1999), *The Health Act*, HMSO, London.

Kingdon, D. (1996), 'Supervision Registers: Caring or Controlling?' *British Journal of Hospital Medicine*, 56, (9), pp. 470-2.

Mental Health Act Commission (1997), $7^{th}$ *Biennial Report 1995-1997*, Department of Health, London.

Mental Health Task Force (1994), *Priorities for Action*, NHS Executive, London.

Patmore, C. and Weaver, T. (1991), *Community Mental Health Teams: Lessons for Planners and Managers*, Report to Department of Health, Good Practices in Mental Health, London.

Sharma, V.K., Wilkinson, G. and Fear, S. (1999), 'Health of the Nation Outcome Scales: A Case Study in General Psychiatry', *British Journal of Psychiatry*, vol. 174, pp. 395-8.

Shaw, J., Appleby, L., Amos, T., McDonnell, R., Harris, C., McCann, K., Bickley, H. and Parsons, R. (1999), 'Mental Disorder and Clinical Care in People Convicted of Homicide: National Clinical Survey', *British Medical Journal*, vol. 318, no. 18, pp. 1240-4.

Taylor, P. and Gunn, J. (1999), 'Homicide by People with Mental Illness: Myth and Reality', *British Journal of Psychiatry*, vol. 174, pp. 9-14.

West, M.A. and Field, R. (1995), 'Teamwork in Primary Health Care. 1 Perspectives from Organisational Psychology', *Journal of Interprofessional Care*, vol. 9, pp. 117-22.

Wing, J.K., Beevor, A.S., Curtis, R.H., Park, S.B.G., Hadden, S. and Burns, A. (1998), 'Health of the Nation Outcome Scales (HONOS). Research and Development', *British Journal of Psychiatry*, vol. 172, pp. 11-18.

White, E. (1990), *The Third Quinquennial National Community Psychiatric Nursing Surveys*, Department of Nursing, University of Manchester, Manchester.

Wooff, K., Goldberg, D. and Fryers, T. (1986), 'Patients in Receipt of Community Psychiatric Nursing Care in Salford 1976 – 1982', *Psychological Medicine*, vol. 16, pp. 407-14.

# 2 Mental Health Inquiries

MAGGIE CLIFTON AND DAVID DUFFY

## Introduction

This chapter reports on an analysis of some 500 recommendations of 42 mental health inquiry reports published between 1990 and July 1997 (see appendix 1). The analysis was carried out by a multi-disciplinary research team (representing nursing, social policy and health service research) with members from the NHS Executive North West Regional Office, Mental Health Services of Salford NHS Trust and Ashworth Hospital Authority. A project Steering Group consisted of senior managers from these agencies. Almost by definition, the recommendations of the inquiry reports were intended to specify targets for quality improvement and were found to be a rich source of expert guidance on what needed to be done to improve mental health services. One of the authors (MC) is both a social scientist, who has published in the area of social policy research, and a general manager who has worked in voluntary sector mental health services. She is currently employed as a Research and Clinical Effectiveness Co-ordinator at Ashworth Hospital Authority. The other author (DD) is a Senior Mental Health Nurse working at Mental Health Services, Salford NHS Trust. He has researched and published extensively on the subject of suicide and self-harm, and has served as a panel member for a number of mental health inquiries.

The chapter begins with the policy context within which mental health inquiries are held and their relevance to targeting in mental health services. This is followed by insights contained in some of the literature that has grown up around the 'inquiry industry', followed by a brief statement of the aims and methodology of the work. Findings are presented and the chapter is concluded by a discussion of the potential value and limitations of these inquiries in improving the quality of services and care to people with severe mental health problems.

## Background to Mental Health Inquiries

Historically, mental health inquiries in the 1960s and 1970s concentrated on allegations of neglect and ill-treatment of hospital patients, whilst most inquiries in the 1990s have been focussed on homicides committed by people with a known history of psychiatric treatment. Since 1994 Government guidance has required that an independent inquiry be held in the case of homicides and other 'serious incidents' in mental health services (DoH, 1994). Between the beginning of 1990 and the first quarter of 1999, 67 inquiry reports had been published, and another 30 had been set in motion. So, when all of these have been completed, nearly 100 reports into homicides and other serious incidents will have been made available for public scrutiny during the decade. Mental health inquiries have now come to be seen as an indicator of failings in the policy and practice of community care (Bennett, 1996; Zito, 1996). Some inquiries have, however, also pointed to areas of good practice that have been commended as models for practice (Blom-Cooper *et al.*, 1995; 1996).

The Government itself recently published *Modernising Mental Health Services* (DoH, 1998), a document which sets out the new national mental health policy agenda. The document acknowledges the limitations of past policies, for example the failure of adult mental health care in the community and the institutionally focused *Mental Health Act* (House of Commons, 1983). The long succession of mental health inquiries sought to highlight such limitations, often through the painstaking investigation of individual tragedies. They also sought to spell out the lessons from their investigations and to recommend good practice that could inform and complement the development of 'safe, sound and supportive' mental health services.

*Insights from the Literature*

Learning from incidents and sharing good practice are both key features of the policy of Clinical Governance. Therefore, by highlighting areas of practice and service delivery for emulation, as well as areas for improvement, mental health inquiries could be seen as contributing data for implementing this policy - within the limitations of the inquiry process.

A number of different and possibly incompatible functions have been identified for homicide and other inquiries. The main purpose of inquiries is to establish the facts leading up to the incident(s), in order to:

- learn from past errors about operational and professional practice and management arrangements, in order to prevent recurrence;
- establish culpable responsibility for what happened; and
- provide explanations and reassurance to relatives, victims, patients and the general public (Lingham and Murphy, 1996).

Despite these generally welcome functions, there is a growing amount of criticisms of the 'inquiry industry' as it currently operates. It has been estimated that the cost of a homicide inquiry lies between £100,000 and £500,000 - excluding the cost of legal representation (*ibid*). Assuming an average cost of £300,000 per inquiry, something in the order of a minimum of £29.1 million has been directed to supporting the 'inquiry industry'. This sort of expenditure can only be justified if the inquiry process is indeed capable of bringing about changes to the provision of services - and therefore of improving the quality of provision. However, a number of further criticisms suggest that this may not necessarily be the outcome of the present inquiry process. These include:

- lack of fairness;
- nature of the evidence;
- focus on the 'rare extremes' of mental illness;
- exclusion of serious incidents other than homicide from mandatory inquiry;
- commissioned by local managers and carried out primarily by legal, health and social care professionals;
- repetition of findings and recommendations; and,
- no requirement for follow up.

Inquiries are mandatory, but not usually statutory. As such, they do not offer any 'procedural or prescriptive rights' and, in their role of establishing culpability, can therefore be criticised as inherently unfair. The reasons for this are that inquiries:

- make no presumption of professional innocence;
- may deliberate in private;
- operate without prescribed and known procedural rules;
- do not provide a right to cross-examination; and,
- do not provide a right of appeal to challenge findings.

Professional bodies should, therefore, be the locus for establishing professional culpability, leaving inquiries to focus on establishing causal explanations (Eastman, 1996). The Zito Trust is committed to the continuation of public, independent inquiries which best service 'the rights of families and significant others who have been bereaved ... and the public interest' (Howlett, 1997, p.6).

The nature of the evidence provided by inquiries is limited to single case studies. Petch and Bradley (1997) argue that inquiring into a single event in a particular service judged by expert opinion fails to establish association, let alone direct causation, between the identified failings of services and professional practice on the one hand, and the homicide or other serious incident, on the other. Indeed Hally (1995, p.9), one of the panel members of the inquiry into the death of Georgina Robinson in Torbay, goes so far as to say that:

> The tragedy at the Edith Morgan Centre was not the result of a unique set of circumstances. Any clinician reading *The Falling Shadow* will recognise situations from their own experience.

One, or even many, inquiries in themselves will not identify why these 'situations' lead to serious incidents in some services, but not in others. Even the Confidential Inquiry approach (Boyd, 1996; Appleby, 1999), considering much larger numbers of cases and looking at both homicide and suicide, does not avoid this limitation. The methodology of looking retrospectively at only those services and situations where things have gone wrong without any form of comparator does not enable causal relationships to be identified, however large the numbers. Alternative responses have been suggested, including a primary focus on local service audit (Eastman, 1996). Petch and Bradley (1997) suggest a large research study to list specific service and practice deficiencies identified by inquiries, followed by an investigation of many services for the presence or absence of those characteristics and their relationship to serious incidents. Possible causative links might then be identified, potentially leading to studies using randomised controlled trials.

Several commentators have highlighted that mandatory inquiries apply only to homicide and not to other forms of serious incident such as suicide or deaths associated with neuroleptic drugs (Davies, 1995; Eastman, 1996). As such the process is limited primarily to one particular type of serious incident. All inquiries do, however, focus attention on the 'rare extremes' of mental disorder (Strong, 1996), with the undesirable consequence of raising the association between mental disorder and violence in the public mind, in the minds of those diagnosed as requiring psychiatric treatment, and of their relatives, friends and employers.

Although independent of the service where the incident(s) occurred, inquiries are mainly commissioned by purchasers of those local services who appoint the chair and members. Panels are primarily composed of health, social care and legal professionals, and can be experienced as a 'cover up' by relatives and voluntary organisations (Davies, 1995). They rarely include service users, although the case for their inclusion is well made (Lindow and Sandford, 1996).

With regard to improving the quality of services, there are several criticisms. The most serious of these concern:

- the recurrence of the same themes and subjects within many inquiry reports;
- failure of the process to require any demonstration by the service in receipt of recommendations that these have been implemented; and,
- the failure of such services to provide any justification for inaction.

The repetition of themes has become a frequent criticism of the inquiry process (Davies, 1995; Eastman, 1996; Kent, 1996; Muijen, 1996). To Strong (1996), this suggests that local services are struggling with similar problems, and that there is a need for national policy makers to address these issues, including the resource implications. In conjunction with the cost, Bennett (1996) suggested that it might be more valuable to put resources into improving services, with more training and consideration of the (then) 300 recommendations already produced. Davies (1996), a member of a number of inquiry panels, reports her experience on being asked by the report's commissioners to revisit the Oxford services investigated after the killing of Jonathan Newby. This indicates that such 're-audit' can be done and proved useful in demonstrating how far the services had gone in improving matters identified in the report - although no doubt making this a mandatory requirement would add appreciably to the cost.

A number of commentators (Eastman, 1996; Muijen, 1996; Howlett, 1997) suggest that a central secretariat for inquiries would assist in streamlining and standardising the process of inquiries, standardising the format of reports and facilitating access to them. This would reduce the cost of inquiries and enable lessons to be learnt more widely than under the present arrangements.

### Aims of the Study

Whilst recognising the limitations of the inquiry method, a small multi-disciplinary team of researchers carried out an analysis of recommendations in 42 inquiry reports (see appendix 1) during 1996/97. The primary aim of this study was to make it easier for all those involved in mental health care to benefit from these intensive and expensive inquiries, and to reduce the risk of repeating mistakes of the past. By this means, the team planned to bring together common themes and issues in an accessible format that would enable the conclusions to be communicated to a wider audience and would facilitate the wider application of inquiry recommendations. This study was intended to complement other work in which themes and issues have been drawn together from mental health inquiry reports. Other studies have focussed on:

- issues from a more limited number of reports (Kent, 1996; Lipsedge and Bland, 1997; MacKay, 1997; Petch and Bradley, 1997);
- specific applications of inquiry reports (Reith, 1997; Duffy *et al.*, 1997); and,
- more limited themes arising from inquiries (Manthorpe, 1998; Reith, 1998; Ward and Applin, 1998).

The Zito Trust has published selected recommendations verbatim without further analysis as a campaigning document (Sheppard, 1995; Sheppard, 1996).

## Methodology

The intention was to draft 'statements' derived from the recommendations of inquiry reports deemed to have relevance for a wider audience, but which remained grounded in the language and concerns of the reports themselves. Inquiry reports were identified from three sources: Peay (1996), Sheppard (1995; 1996), and Institute of Mental Health Law website. Since its creation, the latter source has proved to be particularly valuable because it contains updated lists of published reports and inquiries in progress.

The analysis was restricted to recommendations only; issues raised in the text, but not taken up in the recommendations, were not included. All the recommendations were analysed with the exception of those judged by the researchers as not generalisable to a wider audience. This included those targeted solely on named local bodies (e.g. a trust, health commissioning body, local authority or voluntary organisation); and, those targeted on national or central bodies (e.g. Royal Colleges, Department of Health or Mental Health Act Commission).

Owing to the large volume of written information involved, content analysis was employed. This method examines the language used in communication, and systematically draws out the words or phrases used by the original authors to convey important ideas and concepts. It was used to distil the central themes from each of the reports and to facilitate the development of generalisable summary statements. The first 21 reports were analysed by a team of four. In the first instance three reports were analysed individually and consensus reached on the key themes and sub-themes. Where there were differences of opinion, consensus was reached through discussion. Definitions for each heading and sub-heading were also agreed. Each researcher then independently classified approximately five reports. During this process, regular meetings were held to consider proposed additions to the headings and sub-headings and to resolve any uncertainties. Recommendations were brought together under headings and sub-headings using computer software. Two members of the working group led the process of creating 'summary statements' from these collated recommendations, with support and advice from the other members of the group. The statements were grounded in the recommendations, and no additional subjects were added. A 'critical reader group' was identified representing providers and purchasers of services for people with mental health problems, to assess the clarity, usefulness and relevance of the statements. The statements and their organisation were revised in the light of these comments. The second 21 reports were later analysed by the authors, using the same selection criteria, headings and sub-heading to create statements reflecting the recommendations.

**Findings**

*Identifying Themes*

Table 2.1 lists the main headings identified as a result of the initial analysis of recommendations into themes and sub-themes. In agreeing these headings we aimed to minimise our interpretation of the sense of recommendations by using words and concepts taken from the recommendations wherever possible. Throughout, alphabetical order is used to avoid inferring relative importance of particular issues, which would in practice depend on local circumstances. The Table identifies the *reports* in which the theme occurred and the number of combined *'statements'* that were identified under each theme.

**Table 2.1   Classification of inquiry recommendations**

| Theme | Reports (N) | Statements (N) |
|---|---|---|
| Anti-discriminatory practice | 11 | 9 |
| Care of disturbed patients | 14 | 38 |
| Care Programme Approach | 37 | 90 |
| Communications and confidentiality | 35 | 13 |
| Complaints | 4 | 13 |
| Empowerment | 24 | 33 |
| Incidents and inquiries | 21 | 32 |
| Inter-agency working | 36 | 64 |
| Mental Health Act, 1983 | 20 | 41 |
| Mentally disordered offenders | 6 | 9 |
| Monitoring and audit | 31 | 21 |
| Multi-disciplinary working | 29 | 20 |
| Policies and procedures | 7 | 4 |
| Professional responsibilities | 29 | 44 |
| Records and record-keeping | 27 | 19 |
| Risk assessment and management | 31 | . 36 |

| | | |
|---|---|---|
| Service provision | 30 | 53 |
| Staff development | 33 | 59 |
| Staff management | 26 | 52 |
| Therapeutic approaches | 21 | 26 |

The number (N) of reports and statements appearing under each theme indicates their relative frequency. This analysis confirms the impression that some themes are more common than others - Inter-agency Working, Communications and Confidentiality, the Care Programme Approach, Monitoring and Audit, Risk Assessment and Management, and Staff Development appear in three-quarters of the reports or more. These are closely followed by: Service Provision, Multi-disciplinary Working, Professional Responsibilities, Records and Record-keeping, Staff Management, and Empowerment, identified in over half the reports. Incidents and Inquiries, the Mental Health Act and Therapeutic Approaches are followed by the remaining five headings. The Table also indicates that, in terms of the detail and by our analysis, there was a great deal of differentiation within those broad themes. Even after combining similar recommendations into statements, there were in most cases more statements than reports and in some cases (e.g. Care Programme Approach, Inter-Agency Working, Staff Development) about twice as many statements as reports.

*Recommendations*

The remainder of this section summarises the main contents of each heading and comments on the recommendations in general. Many of the recommendations contained detail relevant to more than one heading and, as far as possible, were included under the one that was judged to be the most substantive theme. In some cases, statements were included under more than one heading. After each summary, one or two examples of the statements generated by the content analysis are provided, which illustrate the level of detail contained within the recommendations.

*Anti-Discriminatory Practice* Recommendations related to equal opportunities, privacy, services for people from ethnic minorities, services for women, the rights of services users and their carers, and the Patient's Charter. Anti-discriminatory practice in human resources management was included. However, not all aspects of anti-discriminatory practice - such as the availability of therapeutic services for patients from ethnic minorities - were mentioned in the recommendations. Example statement:

> There is a clear equal opportunities policy covering in-patient services, which is implemented on the wards and relevant departments of the hospital, and which addresses the issue of racism.

*Care of Disturbed Behaviour* Recommendations were analysed under this heading where the term 'disturbed' was used, where violent or potentially violent behaviour had been specified or implied, and where specific management techniques were the focus of the recommendations. The recommendations covered the need for liaison and communication between agencies and staff, and made reference to use of physical restraint, seclusion, observation, searches, shields, locked wards and the deployment of staff in response to incidents. The recommendations focussed primarily on caring for disturbed patients in in-patient settings. Example statement:

> There are regular clinical audits of the use of special observation and the results are discussed with both medical and nursing staff.

*Care Programme Approach* The Care Programme Approach (CPA) was introduced in 1991 (DoH, 90) and requires health service providers to collaborate with local authority social services providers and other relevant agencies in making arrangements for the care of people with severe mental illness in the community. Although some inquiries were published prior to the introduction of the CPA, some recommendations were incorporated under this heading as being 'in the spirit of' the guidance. The recommendations incorporated into statements for this section focus specifically on meeting the needs of individuals, and follow the progress of a patient from assessment of needs to discharge, or extended leave from hospital care. They are distinguished from those relating to inter-agency working more generally which were analysed under the broader heading.

Many of these recommendations covered similar ground to *Building Bridges* (DoH, 1995) - but this fact indicates that the publication of the document has not in itself prevented further serious incidents linked with failures in collaborative working. Recommendations related to the CPA in general, and highlighted aspects of multi-disciplinary and multi-agency approaches to:

- assessment of a range of needs;
- care planning and the co-ordination of care for both in-patients and clients in community settings;
- co-ordination of transfers within the same service; and,
- planning for and implementing discharge or extended leave.

Interestingly, not all recommendations fully reflected the guidance. For example:

- although there are three levels of the CPA, one recommendation specified only two tiers;
- another recommendation incorporated the notion of a 'night staff key worker' - which conflicts with the principle of a single person with responsibility for co-ordinating care; and,
- although a patient with schizophrenia may properly be subject to level 1 CPA, one recommendation implied that such a diagnosis required level 2 or 3.

Again, none of the recommendations relevant to the CPA incorporated issues of race or culture. Example statements:

There is an agreed protocol for operating the CPA between specialist units and local services, which recognises the joint responsibility.

The GP for any person subject to the CPA is provided with a copy of the care plan and informed of any change to that plan.

*Communications and Confidentiality* Recommendations were made about both inter-agency and intra-agency communications, including communications with users and carers. Policies and procedures to enhance communication and systems for arriving at common agreements and shared understanding were stressed.

The difficult question of maintaining confidentiality of personal information, whilst meeting the legitimate needs of the various players for patient/client information in order to provide an adequate and safe service, was recognised. The need to balance the requirements of confidentiality with those of risk management was highlighted. From another perspective, the importance of sharing agency policies on confidentiality with service users was stressed, as was the value of seeking consent to share information. *The Protection and Use of Patient Information* (DoH, 1997) provides further guidance on this topic. Example statement:

> Staff are aware of the need to share information about patient/client needs and management, balancing the requirements of confidentiality and risk management. There is an over-riding duty to breach confidentiality in the interests of a potential victim.

*Complaints*   Inquiry reports made recommendations on complaints procedures and systems in the NHS, other statutory bodies and the independent sector. Recommendations covered: circumstances in which complaints might need to be referred to the police; the need for prompt investigation; the use of independent investigators; the scope of investigations into complaints; computerised complaints registers; and, policies/guidelines for use across the service. It may be argued that the NHS complaints procedure now addresses many of the concerns raised by the recommendations.  Example statement:

> Outside interviewers are brought in to the investigating team only in exceptional circumstances.

*Empowerment*   Recommendations relating to advocacy, carer and user involvement were coded under this heading. Recommendations included the need for an independent, adequately resourced and competently staffed advocacy service that is ethnically sensitive. There was specific reference to the provision of advocacy for patients subject to Section 117 of the *Mental Health Act* (House of Commons, 1983).

The central value of knowledge provided by relatives, friends and other informal carers to health care professionals was stressed, as were the rights of informal carers to information about services, and to be kept informed about the needs of the patient/client, subject to the latter's consent. Example statement:

> There is an independently managed and adequately resourced patient advocacy service to assist users in expressing their views, which is ethnically

sensitive and staffed by competent personnel. This is available for in-patient and community settings

*Incidents and Inquiries* Support for staff, patients and their relatives in the wake of a serious, untoward incident was recommended. Procedures for reporting and responding to incidents were suggested, as was a requirement for reviewing procedures. Recommendations were made about internal and external inquiries following incidents, including terms of reference, composition of inquiry teams, timing of inquiries, training for those conducting inquiries and the need for co-operation and communication. Example statement:

> After a serious incident the whole multi-disciplinary ward team meets to review all the issues which led to the particular incident.

*Inter-Agency Working* Recommendations covered general issues around inter-agency collaboration, as well as making points about specific agencies and relationships between them. These included NHS commissioners and providers (primary, secondary and tertiary), local authority social services departments, housing providers, the criminal justice system, area child protection services and independent agencies. References were made to:

- liaison arrangements and communications systems;
- policies, procedures and guidelines to support inter-agency working;
- the involvement of service users in promoting collaborative work; and,
- professional roles and responsibilities.

As with the CPA, many of these recommendations cover similar ground to *Building Bridges* (DoH, 1995). Perhaps surprisingly, there is limited reference to child protection. Although child protection issues featured in a number of inquiry reports, only one recommendation was identified which made specific reference to this topic. Example statements:

> There is a shared understanding between all stakeholders in mental health care about their respective contributions to the service and its future pattern,

which enables individual agencies to develop their own strategies in partnership with each other.

Commissioning authorities provide guidelines for general practitioners about the circumstances in which they should be wary of removing mentally ill patients from their lists.

*Mental Health Act, 1983*   Some recommendations were of general relevance to the Act and its application in practice. References were made specifically to proper implementation of Sections 12, 17, 62, 117 and 136 of the Act and to the role and functioning of Approved Social Workers and Mental Health Review Tribunals (House of Commons, 1983). Example statement:

When a patient who is subject to Section 117 aftercare moves from one area to another, a joint case conference is held between those currently providing the aftercare and those in the area to which the patient is moving.

*Mentally Disordered Offenders*   Several recommendations referred to services for mentally disordered offenders and to arrangements for meeting their needs. Reports recommended improvements in working relationships between agencies, sharing information, and in the provision of services required to meet identified needs. There was also specific reference to the role of the 'appropriate adult'. Example statement:

There is a system for ensuring that mentally disordered offenders are only referred to Court in circumstances which are jointly agreed by health services, social services and the police.

*Monitoring and Audit*   Recommendations were made about the review, monitoring and audit of services, policies and procedures. This included general matters such as monitoring caseloads and quality standards. Clinical audit should cover issues relating to patient care and treatment, including uni-disciplinary and multi-disciplinary topics. The inspection of registered homes was also considered. Example statement:

CPN caseloads are reported to management at regular intervals for monitoring purposes and to ensure equitable distribution of caseloads. The nature of each caseload is reviewed in order to give priority to patients with severe and enduring mental health problems.

*Multi-disciplinary Working* - The proper creation and functioning of multi-disciplinary teams and their individual members were central to many recommendations under this heading. This included the allocation of individual members to teams and their responsibilities, as well as methods of working together. Again, issues of record-keeping and information exchange between professionals were raised. Example statement:

> The role of the multi-disciplinary care team and its individual members is clearly defined.

*Policies and Procedures* - Recommendations covered the processes of development, implementation and monitoring of policies, procedures and guidelines in general. These included the central recording of clinical policies and procedures that are in operation and the involvement of staff who will be responsible for implementation in developing policies and procedures. There should be systems to ensure that clinical policies and procedures exist, are consistent internally and with external requirements, and are implemented and monitored. All relevant policies and procedures should be kept in a single file, which is accessible to staff and is indexed, using the same structure for each clinical area. Example statement:

> There is a central register of clinical policies and guideline documents, which records, what documents have been placed on which wards and when.

*Professional Responsibilities* Many recommendations stressed that the role and responsibilities of health care professionals should be clearly identified. They referred to:

- collection of all relevant information relating to client/patient needs;
- access to specialist advice and to appropriate information; and,
- understanding on the part of professionals of their own role, that of others with whom they work and how these interrelate.

Specific reference was made to consultant psychiatrists, including Responsible Medical Officers, junior medical staff, nursing and social work staff, and those taking on the role of key worker. Example statements:

> The 'named nurse' or 'associate nurse' is present at all occasions when decision are being taken as to the future of the patient, including any regular multi-disciplinary team meeting.

> Discharge letters are always approved by a consultant psychiatrist and deal with social aspects of care in addition to the purely medical. Discharge letters written by junior medical staff are monitored.

*Records and Record-Keeping*   Recommendations referred to the recording of information about service users. They referred to technological and management systems for the storage, security, retrieval and disposal of information, and patients' access to their own records. In particular, the importance of record-keeping systems that assure access to appropriate information by the multi-disciplinary team involved in patient care, is a recurring theme.   Specific mention is made of health and social care records, and of the quality of nursing, medical and administrative information. Example statement:

> Providers give consideration to introducing integrated multi-disciplinary notes, which are organised to make essential details easily accessible.

*Risk Assessment and Management*   Inquiry recommendations see effective assessment and management of risk as key issues. Both strategic and operational aspects of reducing risk are reported. Detailed points are made about steps that should be included in risk assessment procedures. These include reference to:

- the risk of harm to self or others;
- indicators of relapse; and,
- sharing risk information between members of care teams and agencies providing care.

This group of recommendations also includes reference to safety in the design of buildings and levels of physical security. Again, the statements are addressed to a range of disciplines and agencies, including statutory providers of health, social care, as well as housing and the independent sector. Example statement:

Where a mentally ill patient has a past history of violence to others, a risk assessment is carried out and recorded prior to discharge, regardless of the presence or absence of other variables such as non-compliance or substance misuse.

*Service Provision*   Many reports made reference to the provision of adequate resources of various types. The recommendations covered strategic (service planning, resource allocation) and operational issues, including the provision of a wide range of:

- general and forensic mental health services;
- other health service provision;
- community services - the full range of accommodation, day, occupational and educational services;
- befriending; and,
- support to informal carers.

Recommendations were addressed to the full range of statutory and independent providers. Enquiry reports considered only those issues leading up to the incident, so there is no reference to balancing conflicting demands, or to working within resource constraints. Local users of these reports would have to decide for themselves what 'adequate' resources implied in their own context. Example statements:

Day care services are provided in: local areas; in premises which reflect ordinary life principles; in groups which reflect common interests; with outreach to enable social integration into the community.

Separate services are provided for patients requiring different levels and types of nursing care, such as:

- patients on acute admission wards;
- patients who are likely to present severe behavioural problems;
- frail elderly mentally infirm patients; and
- young people with substance misuse problems.

*Staff Development*   A common theme was the importance of staff training and development. Recommendations dealt with arrangements for providing, and quality assurance of, development activities. Substantive areas included: supervision and support, CPA training, training about specific disorders, effective induction, staff appraisal, management of violent behaviour, observation, and communication skills. The development of medical, nursing, social work and voluntary sector staff is included. Example statements:

> There is an annual review of the performance, abilities and training needs of all staff.

> Newly appointed health care assistants have an understanding of the needs of clients with whom they will be working prior to commencing work with those clients.

*Staff Management*   Recommendations were made about a wide range of issues in the management of different professionals working in a variety of agencies. There were some points about recruitment and more extensive reference to adequate staffing levels, the deployment of staff, and the provision of proper support to staff. Again, those using these recommendations must interpret 'adequate' in the light of their own circumstances and competing demands on resources. There were no references to the retention of staff and workforce planning, which are undoubtedly important issues. Example statements:

> Particular care is given to the selection of staff who are going to work with elderly, frail individuals.

> Purchasers of social care ensure that there are sufficient forensic social workers to meet local need.

*Therapeutic Approaches*   Recommendations were made about the provision of a range of treatments and therapies, delivered in a variety of settings by different health care professionals. As well as medication, this includes behaviour modification, psychodynamic expertise, occupational therapy, anger management therapy, and therapeutic relationships. The importance of a balanced, needs-led approach to the provision of therapies by adequately skilled personnel is stressed. Example statement:

> There is open debate about the nature and treatment of mental illness, particularly the use of high doses of medication.

**Discussion and Conclusions**

This review of the recommendations of 42 inquiry reports highlights the breadth and range of topics covered. As noted elsewhere, there is much repetition in the broader themes, such as risk assessment, communication, and collaborative working between agencies and disciplines. Given the nature of the inquiry process as single case studies, the extent of repetition of broad themes might indicate either systematic bias on the part of inquiry panels, or a genuine reflection of deep-seated and endemic difficulties and failings in service provision and professional practice. However, the more detailed combined statements indicate that within these broad themes there is much more differentiation, arising from the specific circumstances of the incidents which precipitated the inquiry in the first place. This degree of differentiation within the broader themes suggests to us that inquiry panels are highlighting real and complex issues that should be seen as arising from wider phenomena rather than isolated events.

The interrelated nature of these themes indicates that whole service systems need to be considered for improvement, not just individual topics such as risk assessment or staff training. Looking at individual topics in isolation from each other, and from the rest of the system, might improve that single area, but will have limited impact on the functioning of the service as a whole. Continuous quality improvement needs to take place within the context of a coherent framework, such as the Excellence Model (British Quality Foundation, undated).

Whilst the inquiries rightly focus primarily on what has gone wrong prior to a serious incident, there are occasions when good practice is commended. Particular examples of this are the promotion in *The Falling Shadow* of the history taken by a senior registrar in Broadmoor (Blom-Cooper *et al.*, 1995), and the commendation of a report produced by an Occupational Therapy Technical Instructor (Blom-Cooper *et al.*, 1996).

Clinical Governance and clinical effectiveness require evidence-based practice and service delivery. However, the evidence of inquiries is simply accumulated expert opinion, and regardless of the number of inquiries and the similarities between their findings, this evidence will never become a substitute for scientific research. As well as being the product of single case studies, inquiry recommendations are only ever based on hindsight. This means that there can be no certainty that, if things had been as recommended prior to the inquiry, that the events under investigation, or something very similar, would still not have happened. Similar reservations apply to the Confidential Inquiries (Boyd, 1996; Appleby *et al.*, 1999) even though they deal with much larger numbers.

Within the context of the quality agenda and Clinical Governance, inquiry reports surely have a role to play. In mental health, the scientific evidence-base for both treatments and service models is limited. The use of alternative sources of information for continuous quality improvement is expected in the policy literature - and this includes learning from incidents on the one hand, and from good practice on the other. Whilst an isolated example, it should be noted that the trigger for one inquiry was a homicide followed by suicide, in which the perpetrator had *not* been assessed as suffering from serious mental illness.

Inquiry reports might be of more value to the wider service if there were a separation of functions. It has been argued elsewhere on the grounds of fairness that demonstrating professional culpability sits uneasily with establishing the facts in order to improve services. Perhaps it might also make for more effective inquiries if these two functions were separated, as the most appropriate format for investigations of fact is not necessarily the most appropriate for establishing culpability.

Whilst it might not be cost-effective to require inquiry panels to return, after say a year, to evaluate action in response to their recommendations, service managers could be expected to give account of how they have responded. This does not preclude services not implementing change on the basis of inquiry recommendations, but managers and practitioners would be expected to justify such a decision. Where recommendations have been accepted, a prioritised and timetabled action plan with a note of outcomes achieved could be required. Such a mechanism would satisfy the demand of Clinical Governance for 'continuous quality improvement' - rather than simply a 'one-off' response to homicides and serious incidents. A central co-ordinating function ensuring a standard approach to inquiries and their reports, and which would also be a single point of distribution would enable inquiry reports to contribute to quality improvement more widely than simply the service in which they originated.

Homicides and other serious incidents that give rise to inquiries are clearly tragedies for those individuals directly involved. The continuing number of inquiries being published and in process suggests that there are systematic difficulties in providing adequate services in this very complex field. Whilst there are those who have seen the increasing number of inquiries as indicating that 'community care has failed', we should not forget the number of inquiries in the 1960s and 1970s which, at least in part, contributed to the conclusion that institutional care had failed. As others have noted, a number of deaths have arisen from the use of neuroleptic drugs (Davies, 1995), and adverse events have been associated with the use of seclusion (Fisher, 1994). Whilst it is incumbent on all involved to make every effort to minimise the risk of serious incidents, there is a danger that an over-cautious approach to risk assessment and management will contribute to increasing numbers of 'false positives'. In this situation, people remain in more restrictive environments than necessary - but those errors of judgement will not come to light.

Whatever models of care have been adopted it is clear that mental health care, particularly for those with serious mental illness, is not a risk-free business. Providing a quality service, which minimises risk without unnecessary restriction, will always be a complex task with the potential for errors of judgement and service failures. Inquiry recommendations tell us 'what' to do but shed little light on 'how' to do it. The continuing stream of reports suggests that it is easier to write recommendations than to implement them. In these circumstances, however, no-one can be complacent and all information of potential value should be drawn upon. Despite the limitations of the inquiry process, these reports and their recommendations offer one source of information that can aid self-critical reflection by commissioners and providers, and thus contribute to continuous quality improvement. The fact that inquiry recommendations are grounded in specific, concrete events and are informed by expert knowledge lends them a weight and credibility which is of great potential value in making decisions about the targeting of areas for quality improvement.

## References

Appleby, L., Shaw, J. and Amos, T. (1999), *Safer Services: National Confidential Inquiry into Suicide and Homicide by People with Mental Illness,* Department of Health, London.

Bennett, D. (1996), 'Homicide, Inquiries and Scapegoating', *Psychiatric Bulletin,* vol.20, pp. 298-300.

British Quality Foundation (undated), *Guide to the Business Excellence Model,* British Quality Foundation, London.

Davies, N. (1996), 'An Inquiring Mind', *Mental Health Nursing,* vol. 16, no. 5, pp. 4-5.

Davies, R. (1995), 'Inquiry into Inquiries', *OpenMIND* 75, June/July, pp. 6-8.

Department of Health (1990), *Health and Social Services Development: "Caring for People" The Care Programme Approach for People with a Mental Illness referred to the Special Psychiatric Services,* Joint Health and Social Services Circular, HC(90)23/LASSL(90)11, Department of Health, London.

Department of Health (1994), *Guidance on the Discharge of Mentally Disordered People and their Continuing Care in the Community,* HSG (94) 27, Department of Health, London.

Department of Health (1995), *The Health of the Nation: Building Bridges - A Guide to Arrangements for Inter-agency Working for the Care and Protection of Severely Mentally Ill People,* HMSO, London.

Department of Health (1997), *The Protection and Use of Patient Information,* Guidance, Department of Health, London.

Department of Health (1998), *Modernising Mental Health Services,* The Stationery Office, London.

Duffy, D., Clifton, M. and Dale, C. (1997), 'Mental Health Inquiry Reports: The Lessons for Nursing', *Mental Health Practice,* vol. 2, no. 1, pp. 11-16.

Eastman, N. (1996), 'Inquiry into Homicides by Psychiatric Patients: Systematic Audit Should Replace Mandatory Inquiries', *British Medical Journal,* vol. 311, pp. 1069-71.

Fisher, W.A. (1994), 'Restraint and Seclusion: a Review of the Literature', *The American Journal of Psychiatry,* 151, pp. 1584-91.

Hally, H. (1995), 'Shining a Light into the Shadowlands', *Mental Health Nursing,* vol. 15, no. 2, pp. 7-9.

Howlett, M. (1997), *The Management of Independent Inquiries into Homicides and Serious Incidents of Violence by the Mentally Ill,* Zito Trust, London.

House of Commons (1983), *The Mental Health Act,* HMSO, London.

Institute of Mental Health Law, *Mental Health Inquiries,* http://www.imhl.com.

Kent, I. (1996), 'Reporting Back', *Community Care,* 22-28 February 1996, pp.18-19.

Lindow, V. and Sandford, T. (1996), 'Letter' *Health Service Journal,* 14 November 1996, p. 20.

Lingham, R. and Murphy, E. (1996), 'Deadly Serious', *Health Service Journal,* 31 October 1996, pp. 22-3.

Lipsedge, M. and Bland, S. R. (1997), 'Review of 11 Independent Inquiries into Homicide by Psychiatric Patients, *Clinical Risk,* vol. 3, pp. 171-7.

MacKay, J. (1997), 'Mental Health Inquiries: Learning from Experience', *Mental Health Nursing,* vol. 17, no. 6, pp. 13-6.

Manthorpe, J. (1998), 'Learning Through Inquiry', *Journal of Mental Health,* vol. 7, no. 1, pp. 1-7.

Muijen, M. (1996), 'Heresy About the Inquisitions', *Health Service Journal,* 29 February 1996, p. 25.

Muijen, M. (1997), 'Inquiries: Who Needs Them?', (Editorial) *Psychiatric Bulletin,* 21, pp. 132-3.

Murphy, E. (1996), 'Letter', *Health Service Journal,* 14 March 1996, p. 22.

Petch, E. and Bradley, C. (1997), 'Learning the Lessons from Homicide Inquiries: Adding Insult to Injury?' *Journal of Forensic Psychiatry,* vol. 8, no. 1, pp.161-84.

Peay, J. (ed) (1996), *Inquiries After Homicide,* Duckworth, London.

Reith, M. (1997), 'Mental Health Inquiries: Implications for Probation Practice', *Probation,* vol. 44, no. 2, pp. 66-70.

Reith, M. (1998), 'Risk Assessment and Management: Lessons from Mental Health Inquiry Reports', *Medicine, Law and Society,* vol. 38, no. 3, pp. 221-6.

Sheppard, D. (1995), *Learning the Lessons: Mental Health Enquiry Reports Published in England and Wales between 1969 and 1994. Recommendations for Improving Practice,* The Zito Trust, London.

Sheppard, D. (1996), *Learning the Lessons,* 2nd Edition, The Zito Trust, London.

Strong, S. (1996), 'On the Brink of Disaster', *Community Care,* 22-28 February 1996, pp. 16-7.

Ward, M. and Applin, C. (1998), *The Unlearned Lesson: The Role of Alcohol and Drug Misuse in Homicides Perpetrated by People with Mental Health Problems,* Wynne Howard Books, London.

Zito, J. (1996), 'Letter', *Health Service Journal,* 14 March 1996, p. 22.

## Appendix 1: Inquiry reports: recommendations analysed

*Report of the Independent Panel of Inquiry into the Treatment and Care of Paul Smith* (1997), North West Anglia Health Authority, Peterborough.

*Bolton Hospitals NHS Trust - Independent External Review into Mental Health Services* (1997), Bolton Hospitals NHS Trust, Bolton.

*Report of the Independent Inquiry Team into the Care and Treatment of Martin Mursell* (1997), Camden and Islington Health Authority, London.

*Report of the Independent Inquiry Team - presented to Bromley HA, SE London Probation Service and Bromley SSD* (1997), Bromley Health Authority, Hayes.

*Report of the Inquiry into the Care and Treatment of Darren Carr* (1997), Berkshire Health Authority, Reading.

*Report of the Independent Inquiry into the Care and Treatment of Peter Richard Winship* (1997), Nottingham Health Authority, Nottingham.

*Report of the Inquiry into the Events Leading to the Death of David Howell* (1997), Birmingham Health Authority, Birmingham.

*Report of the Independent Inquiry Team into the Care and Treatment of Gilbert Kopernik-Steckel* (1997), Croydon Health Authority, Croydon.

*Report of the Independent Panel of Inquiry into the Circumstances Surrounding the Absconsion of Trevor Holland from the Care of Horizon NHS Trust on 29th August 1996* (1997), Horizon NHS Trust, Radlett.

*Report of the Inquiry into the Care and Treatment of 5 Individual Patients by Oldham NHS Trust Mental Health Services Commissioned by West Pennine Health Authority* (1997), West Pennine Health Authority, Oldham.

*Report to Northumberland Health Authority into the Care and Treatment of Richard Stoker* (1996), Northumberland Health Authority, Morpeth, Northumberland.

*Report of the Independent Inquiry into the Circumstances Surrounding the Deaths of Robert and Muriel Viner* (1996), Dorset Health Commission, Ferndown.

*Report of the Independent Inquiry into Team into the Care and Treatment of Nilesh Gadher* (1996), Ealing, Hammersmith and Hounslow Health Authority, London.

*Report of the Independent Inquiry into the Care and Treatment of Francis Hampshire* (1996), Redbridge and Waltham  Forest Health Authority, Ilford, Essex.

*Report of the Inquiry into the Care and Treatment of Shaun Armstrong* (1996), Tees Health Authority, Middlesborough.

*Report of the Inquiry into the Care and Treatment of Raymond Sinclair* (1996), West Kent Health Authority, Aylesford.

*Report of the Independent Inquiry Team into the Care and Treatment of Kumbi Mabota* (1996), Redbridge and Waltham Forest Health Authority, Ilford, Essex.

*Caring for the Carer - Report of the Inquiry into the Care of Keith Taylor* (1996), Tees Health Authority, Middlesborough.

*Report into 7 Unexpected Deaths and One Serious Incident of Self-Harm between January 1994 and January 1996* (1996), West Cheshire NHS Trust, Chester.

*Report into the Care of Anthony Smith* (1996), Southern Derbyshire Health, Derby.

*Learning Lessons: Report into the Events Leading to the Incident at St. John's Way Medical Centre in December 1995* (1996), Camden and Islington Health Authority, London.

*Report of the Independent Inquiry Team into the Care and Treatment of Richard John Burton* (1996), Leicestershire Health Authority, Leicester.

Blom-Cooper, L. QC, Grounds, A., Guianan, P., Parker, A. and Taylor, M.  *The Case of Jason Mitchell: Report of the Independent Panel of Inquiry* (1996), Duckworth, London.

Boyd W. *Report of the Confidential Inquiry into Homicides and Suicides by Mentally Ill People* (1996), Royal College of Psychiatrists, London.

*Report of the Inquiry into the Care and Treatment of Philip McFadden* (1995), Scottish Office, Edinburgh.

*The Cooper Inquiry* (1995), Bedfordshire Health Authority, Luton.

Blom-Cooper, L., Hally, H. and Murphy, E. (1995), *The Falling Shadow: One Patient's Mental Health Care 1978-1993,* Duckworth, London.

*Report of the Panel of Inquiry into the Circumstances Surrounding the Deaths of Eileen and Alan Boland* (1995), North West London Mental Health NHS Trust. London.

*The Woodley Team Report: Report of the Independent Review Panel to East London and the City Health Authority and Newham Council, Following a*

*Homicide in July 1994 by a Person Suffering with a Severe Mental Illness* (1995), East London and the City Health Authority and Newham Council, London.

*Report of the Inquiry into the Circumstances Leading to the Death of Jonathan Newby* (1995), Oxfordshire Health Authority, Oxford.

*The Report of the Inquiry into the Care and Treatment of Christopher Clunis* (1994), NE Thames and SE Thames Regional Health Authorities, London.

*Report of the Independent Panel of Inquiry Examining the Case of Michael Buchanan* (1994), North West London Mental Health NHS Trust, London.

*North West London Mental Health Services Inquiry* (1994), North West London Mental Health Services NHS Trust, London.

*Report of the Committee of Inquiry in to theDeath in Broadmoor Hospital of Orville Blackwood and a Review of the Deaths of Two Other Afro-Caribbean Patients 'Big, Black and Dangerous'* (1993), Special Hospital Services Authority, London.

*Review of Deaths Amongst Patients of Oxfordshire Health Authority Mental Health Unit 1990-1991* (1994), Oxfordshire Health Authority, Oxford.

*Report of the Committee of Inquiry into Complaints about Ashworth Hospital* (1992), HMSO, London.

*Report of the Independent Inquiry into Kevin Rooney* (1992), North Thames Regional Health Authority, London.

*Report of the Investigation into Serious Incidents Occurring at the Shrodells Psychiatric Unit, October 1989-November 1990* (1992), SW Hertfordshire Health Authority, St Albans.

*Regional Fact Finding Inquiry into the Admission, Care, Treatment and Discharge of Carol Barratt* (1991), Trent Regional Health Authority, Sheffield.

*Report of the Panel of Inquiry Appointed by the West Midlands RHA to Investigate the Case of Kim Kirkman* (1991), West Midlands Regional Health Authority, Birmingham.

*Report of the Inquiry into the Circumstances Leading to the Death in Broadmoor Hospital of Joseph Watts on 23rd August 1988* (1991), Special Hospital Services Authority, London.

*Report of the Panel of Inquiry Appointed by the North Staffordshire Health Authority to Investigate the Circumstances of the Death of Mrs Alma Simpson on 6th June 1988* (1990), West Midlands Regional Health Authority, Birmingham.

## Acknowledgements

The authors wish to acknowledge the contribution of the NHS Executive North West, Mental Health Services of Salford NHS Trust and Ashworth Hospital Authority, who provided the support, guidance and resources which made the project both possible and enlightening.

# 3 'Serious Mental Illness' – The Language of Moral Panic

WILLIAM SPENCE

## Introduction

Throughout the 1990s, the dominant theme in the media's reporting of incidents involving people deemed to be 'seriously mentally ill', was that mental disorder and violence are linked. The association between violence and mental disorder is not new, and can be traced back to ancient Greece and Rome, where mental disorder was characterised by aimless wandering and violence (Rosen, 1968). The inadequacies of community care mean that the perceived link between mental disorder and violence poses a significant danger to the public. The response of the government to these examples of poor practice and perceived threat has been that services should 'target' people with 'serious mental illness'. This can be seen as an exercise in 'mediating political concern' (Barker *et al.*, 1998). However, targeting this group of people may partially conceal the very real difficulties faced by those who have not acquired the 'serious mental illness' label (Bowers, 1997), and who form the majority of people with mental health needs. This surely requires that a 'significant denial mechanism' (Barker *et al.*, 1998) is employed to exclude the less 'seriously mentally ill' who, until recently, have been deemed deserving of mental health service intervention.

This chapter aims to explore the use of language in relation to those experiencing enduring disorder - as they will be referred to here – and those who purport to help them, together with the contextual factors that give meaning to this discourse. The chapter begins with a discussion of the propensity for language to shape reality in relation to this group, and the now widespread acceptance of the targeting initiative. Then, the disease model of mental illness, and the link between violence and mental illness, will be examined. Next, in line with the contextual constructionist position used in the analysis of social phenomena (Thomson, 1998), the evidence for the apparent over-exaggeration of the risk of violence presented by this group will be briefly considered, and the media hyperbole debunked to some degree. Lastly, the concept of moral panic will be discussed in

75

relation to this group, and several theoretical positions will be used in offering some analysis of its cause in this decade and context. The significance of the lack of opposition to this targeting manoeuvre by the ruling elite of mental health services will be conceded, as will psychiatry's strengthened grip of mental health services, and the increased power of the biomedical model.

## Language, Post Modernism and 'Serious Mental Illness'

The terms 'serious mental illness' and 'severe and enduring mental illness' seem to be increasingly used in an interchangeable fashion by mental health professionals. The implication that mental illnesses which are not enduring, are not severe, will be offensive to many, not least the people who are disabled by 'non-severe' or 'non-serious' disorders. The reductionist assumptions often witnessed in the practice of psychiatry, where preoccupation seems to exist with the chemical alteration of the availability of brain neurotransmitters, are reflected in the term 'serious mental illness'. In this term, the legitimate metaphorical use of the term 'illness' is often replaced by its literal counterpart. The use of such highly medicalised terminology to describe experience will, for many, sound authoritative.

The technocratic nature of the term 'serious mental illness' implies that its conceptualisation is underpinned by a scientific rationale, akin to that often assumed to underpin the diagnostic criteria in use today e.g. *ICD 10* (WHO, 1992) and *DSM IV* (APA, 1994). The use of such classificatory systems may constitute an illusion of freedom from human values and interpretation, while contributing to the technical rationality which undermines the metaphysics of human relationships and experience (Horkheimer, 1972). The patient's reality may be diametric to any diagnostic label. The frailty of humanity is symbolised in this 'reality' by the practice differences amongst practitioners, including medical practitioners, and the cultural influences on the nature of mental disorder, and the language and diagnostic criteria used. Certainly, the use of this term, as the language of modern day psychiatry, cannot be assumed to represent some kind of empirical reality. Indeed, the term 'serious mental illness' is at odds with the prevailing diagnostic classificatory system in Britain, *ICD 10*, where it is simply not recognised. This system adopts the less contentious, if not ideal , term 'disorder' to describe such experiences. While this term rather disappointingly implies that all significant mental health problems may be seen as resulting in some kind of mental chaos, regardless of the environmental chaos which might have provoked them, it may be seen as less reductionist and medical in tone than the term 'serious mental illness'.

When a classificatory scheme is used in conjunction with clinical instruments and other technical protocols in reaching a diagnosis, only someone who would risk being known as unscientific or biased would challenge such a diagnosis (Pardeck and Murphy, 1993). The use of such schemes constitutes a technical operation into which judgements are transformed to create the illusion of objectivity (Dreyfus and Dreyfus, 1986). Valid knowledge, in this instance the diagnosis with its implications for treatment, cannot be expected to simply merge as a consequence of removing human judgement from clinical initiatives (Matarazzo, 1986), (even if this were possible, and it certainly is not possible) in the application of these schemes of classification.

Those who emphasise the reductionist paradigm in mental health care seek to establish a knowledge that is not contaminated by subjectivity. If interpretation can be 'purged from the knowledge acquisition process', then it is assumed that it will be possible to reach this reality (Murphy, 1989, p. 62). This reality is seen to be independent of human action and, to some extent, superior to that which is tainted by human interpretation. It is thus a seductive star to be followed by those struggling in the 'swamp' of practice (Schon, 1991), where few definitive answers exist to the human problems presented to, and by, clients. These overtones have contributed to the tendency for other epistemologies to be overlooked in a policy world where the randomised controlled trial is seen as some kind of gold standard in objectivity. The faith thus associated with scientific method in psychiatry may have contributed to the acceptance of the term 'serious mental illness' with little discussion around its validity or utility.

The medical model locates the source of psychopathology in the individual, and it follows that such an individualist approach should not consider too weightily the cultural factors that constitute the backdrop to the stage of mental phenomena. The field of psychiatry seems to have avoided the overtures of encroaching postmodernism, arguably because of the institutionalised power of psychiatrists and other staff groups who collude with this. Postmodernism in Europe is that period which began with the end of world war one (Denzin, 1991). The failure of the Western intellectual tradition, including the empirical tradition of scientific method and the prevailing Western philosophical tradition of this period, to safeguard civilisation from this unsavoury aspect of human nature, provoked a rethink. The modern perspective on knowledge, as the route to enabling the definition and systematisation of reality with a view to judging it (*ibid*), gave way to an altered view of knowledge. Some philosophers recognised their own participation in creating knowledge (Berger and Luckman, 1966). This was a radical departure from the understanding that the search for knowledge was a search for some kind of purely objective knowledge and information about things. The postmodern focus turned to the process of knowledge acquisition, rather than the product of it (Brennan, 1995). Because our understanding of the process of knowledge acquisition is so immature, we must rely on the discovery of part of a relative truth or knowledge by engaging in conversation in which each participant must enter the world of the other in an attempt to understand it. Few would argue that this is the *modus operandum* of modern day psychiatry, and more might wonder about the motivation of psychiatry to eschew the egalitarianism necessitated by such an approach.

Reality and language have more often been seen as quite distinct entities, although from the post modernist perspective, language may be seen as having the capacity to shape reality. Speech is not thought to 'indicate', 'point to' or 'stand for' something empirical (Mitchell, 1986). It may only be seen as a representation of a more fundamental source of information which is believed to exist. The truth about clients' experience of debilitating disorders is derived from language, and not reality (Lacan, 1977; cited in Murphy, 1989). The language that is used to communicate the client's experience, and the professional discourse which is used to conceptualise this, is used by all to establish a reality which is the focus of therapy. The use of the term 'serious mental illness' may shape this reality in a way which is not conducive to a holistic approach to health or full respect for the client's personal autonomy. Other client groups are here marginalised in the care arena, and there is a risk that progressive practice associated with the care of client groups with stronger advocacy will not be transferred to those experiencing enduring disorder. The language of psychiatry in relation to this group may be seen as a metanarrative of which Lloytard (1984) has expressed some scepticism. This scepticism relates to the way these grand narratives are employed to represent a knowledge base that is used to justify order, but which is not 'embroiled in the contingencies that are part of daily life' (Murphy, 1989, p.61). The language of psychiatry is, perhaps deliberately, far removed from the everyday lives upon which it attempts to impose order. Further, it remains beyond the reach of most of those who may wish to express their distress, or negotiate their care with the people who use it. Cardinal (1996, p103) illustrates this difficulty most vividly in her description of her experience of mental distress:

> Prostrate as I was, withdrawn into my own universe, how to find the words which would flow between us? How to construct the bridge which would join the intense to the calm, the clear to the obscure, which could span this sewer, this river filled with decomposing matter, this treacherous current of fear, that separated the doctor and me, the others and me?

The social, environmental and economic realities of the patient and doctor may be very different and difficult for either to reconcile as the language used to communicate these is changing more rapidly than psychiatry.

Indeed, language is constantly expanding and, therefore, the meaning of reality becomes more difficult to understand. The introduction of the term 'serious mental illness' may represent an acknowledgement of this expansion, and a reaction to it, where the complexities and diversity in client experiences of mental disorder are overly simplified in this meaninglessly over-ambitious umbrella term. If mental disorder is seen as a difference between languages and perceptions of reality, the introduction of a new language of poorly defined technocratic terms will only weaken the linguistic bonds between practitioners and clients. That 'there is no escape from the uncertainty spawned by language' (*ibid.*, p.64) will come as no surprise, or comfort, to policy makers intent on rationing resources to fund services which clearly demonstrate improved outcome for distinct client groups thought to be deserving of the investment. This, however, is a deeply flawed rationale for the introduction of new terms into an already jargon ridden field, which seems to be based more on political expediency than anything which will help practitioners assist clients in understanding the experience of mental disorder.

Because reality is sustained linguistically, it is inadvisable to target mental health interventions at the reintegration of clients into society (*ibid*). The post-modern focus involves the direction of mental health services to the client's experience, which itself is the creation of language. Attention should be paid to this linguistic world as a source of information which may be used in enabling clients' deeper understanding of their experience. The challenge for services is to transcend the current modernist position of psychiatry which views clients as passive recipients whose experiences require to be controlled by its science. This is marked by 'closing, abstraction and distancing of peoples' subject and object characteristics and must move to 'openness, involvement and participation' (White and

Hellerich, 1992, p. 86), in order that further client alienation is obviated and genuine empowerment becomes a goal.

The importance of language in mental health care extends beyond the consideration that it is politically correct. It is central to the therapeutic relationship in defining the clients' experience of mental disorder where this is seen as the appropriate focus of intervention for those caring for this group.


## The Disease Model

The use of the term 'serious mental illness' implies that a disease process is at work. This connotation lends authority to the term and those who use it (Pardeck and Murphy, 1993). The insistence that the technical treatment preferred by the medical profession with this client group, for example, the use of anti-psychotic medication, assumes precedence over lower technology treatments, is typical of our age. The assumption that natural laws govern all our existence fuels the search for these rules, and this is considered the hall mark of *bona fide* science (Murphy, 1989). This has led to those who follow this path being accused of 'symbolic violence' (Thomson, 1984). This author asserts that the disease model promotes 'symbolic violence' because it undermines one form of reality, the patient's lived experience of mental disorder, by a supposedly superior and value free form of reality embodied in the methodology of science.

For some researchers, this may be entirely appropriate where schizophrenic disorder is viewed essentially as a biological illness (Gournay, 1994). This overly simplistic interpretation reflects the dualism that pervades the Western intellectual tradition. The assumed causal links between brain physiology and chemistry and behaviour are predicated on the acceptance of dualism. The search for the effects of natural laws on the brain and behaviour is thought to be truly scientific. However, the disease model has not proved to be particularly fruitful in explaining this phenomenon. The fact that it is necessary to creatively interpret the findings and observations of such scientific studies weakens the claims for the existence of the causal relationships that are enthusiastically sought by medical researchers. As long ago as 1972, Foucault pointed out the foolishness of the natural, rather than the symbolic, treatment of physiological phenomena thought to underpin 'serious mental illness' according to the disease model. He highlighted the need for practitioners to interpret the type of health problem presented, the symptoms presented, and the prognosis. He asserted that any disease constitutes a discursive formation, that is, the use of different statements referring to the same object, which support a strategy or political pattern. Furthermore, he argued that in the case of disease, this discursive formation is one in which the interpretation of evidence is central to the doctor's role. This perspective is particularly indicated here, where the fairly widely accepted stress-vulnerability model (Neuchterlein and Dawson, 1984), highlights the extent of the social and environmental variables implicated in relapse for those experiencing schizophrenia.

**Violence**

The mechanistic imagery presupposed by causality is readily maintained by the modern positivist approach of psychiatry. The causal metaphor is widely applied to the association between mental disorder and violence in the eye of the public. However, in assessing the contribution of mental disorder to the risk of violence there are many variables that form part of a complex social reality. A result of this complexity is that the notion of a causal connection may be almost meaningless. The search for it, via overly simplistic assessment mechanisms and instruments, may be conducted at the expense of the richness of information available which evidences these variables, and which will lead to a more accurate assessment of the risk posed.

This link between mental disorder and violence is both well established and important. It can be seen to drive the formal laws and policies which attempt to control those experiencing mental disorder and, more frequently, enduring disorder, and it determines our informal responses and patterns of interaction with these groups (Monahan, 1992). There can be no doubt that in a number of incidents mental disorder has been tragically linked to violence, and that these tragedies have inspired a reaction from policy makers which has seldom been thought to be warranted (see Appendix 1). There is a long established understanding of the public's perception of the high levels of violence risk presented by those experiencing mental disorder (Deutsch, 1949; Westermeyer and Kroll, 1978; Murphy, 1976; Pescosolido *et al.*, 1999). The study of this linkage poses many methodological problems that has undermined the quality of available evidence and contributed to the weakness of studies in this area (Table 3.1).

**Table 3.1  Methodological weaknesses in the study of the risk of violence presented by those experiencing mental disorder**

- Indicators of violent acts perpetrated by this group in the community are notoriously poor. Records of arrest are almost certainly underestimates as are rates of re-hospitalisation that may only serve to identify those most vulnerable to this behaviour. Self-report of violent acts may also be an underestimate as a result of interviewees wishing to present themselves as positively as possible to the interviewer.

- Given that these indicators are usually weak, then it is surprising that few studies include descriptive information to facilitate the understanding of violence in context (Steadman *et al.*, 1998).

- In relation to contextual factors, few studies report on the timing of violent acts despite the salience of this factor to the delivery of interventions.

- Several studies have included only those who present a predictably high risk of violence, thus limiting the generalisability of these studies to the wider group of sufferers of enduring disorder.

- Social conditions and themes are thought to be exogenous and are often inadequately considered.

- Those experiencing mental disorder may be more likely to be apprehended, or simply give themselves up to the authorities (Robertson, 1988).

These weaknesses are paralleled by the difficulties that practitioners face in predicting dangerousness. Mental health professionals have been found to be wrong in around 90% of attempts (Ennis and Emery, 1978). Monahan and Steadman (1983) reviewed over 200 studies on the association between crime and mental disorder and concluded that this link can be accounted for largely by the demographic and historical characteristics shared by the two populations. When the variables of age, gender, race, social class and previous institutionalisation are controlled, the relationship between crime and mental disorder tends to disappear. However, these assumptions have been questioned by one of the original authors, as social class and previous institutionalisation are highly related to mental disorder (Monahan, 1992). Mental disorder may result in social class decline for sufferers and may be a cause or consequence of mental disorder. Also, if mental disorder causes violence and institutionalisation, then controlling for this will obscure the relationship between these two variables. Nevertheless, many authors have noted mental disorder to be a significant risk factor for violence (Steadman *et al.*, 1998; Bloom, 1989; Wessely and Taylor, 1991), although as Monahan (1992, p.519) points out:

> none of the data give any support to the sensationalised caricature of the mentally disordered served up by the media...Clearly mental health status makes at best a trivial contribution to the overall level of violence in society.

However, this risk is greatly increased where substance misuse coexists with another mental disorder diagnosis (Steadman *et al.*, 1998). These authors demonstrated that at 1-year post discharge follow-up, some 17.9% of those who had experienced 'major mental disorder' but who did not misuse substances, committed violent acts towards others. Some 32.7% of this group were found to have committed other aggressive acts in this post-discharge period. Where substance misuse is implicated in this client group the respective figures increase to 31.1% and 33.7% (Steadman *et al.*, 1998). The methodological problems associated with this study, where patients were compared with other individuals from the same neighbourhood, partly indicate the early stage researchers are at in unravelling the link between mental disorder and violence. Acceptance of these pointers may go some way in opening up a frank and honest debate about the management of the risks posed by this client group when discharged to community care.

## Moral Panic

The first published references to moral panic can be traced to the early 1970s descriptions of the increase in illicit substance misuse and the competition between mods and rockers (Young, 1971; Cohen, 1972). The polemical nature of moral panic, as promulgated in the media, is frequently paralleled in the literature discussion of it, given the dearth of rigorous research in this area. This may well, in turn, be a result of the complex multifactorial nature of the phenomenon's roots. Despite the variety of perspectives on the development of moral panic, general agreement appears to exist on two aspects (Thomson, 1998). Firstly, high levels of concern about the behaviour of a particular group or category of people must be evident. This is exemplified by the concerns expressed by many groups across the 1990s about the risk of violence posed by the recipients of community mental health care. Secondly, a level of hostility towards the group or category viewed as a threat is required. This might be less straightforward to disentangle from the background levels of stigma encountered by those experiencing enduring mental disorder. Perhaps not surprisingly, this media hostility is experienced in a negative manner by some service users as exemplified by the following quote:

> I have a diagnosis of schizophrenia and I am just a normal decent law abiding citizen, non violent and I just try to get on with my life as best I can within the community and these attacks by the press on me are not helping me to do that (Radio 4, 18th April 1995, as cited in Philo, 1996, p.112).

The concerns posed by the risk presented by those experiencing 'serious mental illness' in the community indicate some degree of proportionality (Goode and Ben-Yehuda, 1994) where these may be seen as justifiable to some degree. Waddington (1986) has noted that this is not always the case where concerns may be completely unjustified. Nevertheless, he describes a series of indicators of proportionality that have some relevance to 'serious mental illness'.

Firstly, the exaggeration of statistics may be employed to disproportionately represent a kernel of truth central to the moral panic. Gournay's 1994 claim that 'CPN [community psychiatric nursing] teams were abandoning their work with 'serious mental illnesses' in order to work with people with minor psychiatric disorders in primary health care settings' belies the profoundly disabling effect of these 'minor disorders' on the lives of those experiencing them (Bowers 1997). Similarly, the use of emotive language to describe the situation might be seen as a method of exaggeration. For example, Gournay (1994) describes the extrapolated percentage of those experiencing 'serious mental illness' who were not on the caseload of a mental nurse working in the community to be 'scandalous'. Further exaggeration is implied in McFadyen and Farrington's (1996, p.922) immoderate tones where 'neglect, suicide, violence and murder' associated with mental disorder are seen to 'represent the tip of the iceberg'. They further claim that this should be borne in mind when the media's 'alarmist interpretation' of these incidents is considered by those 'attaching even a moderate amount of scepticism' to it.

Secondly the fabrication of statistics may contribute to disproportionality. This was clearly evidenced in the media's response to the preliminary report of the *Confidential Inquiry into Homicides and Suicides by Mentally Ill People* (Confidential Inquiry, 1994). In his 1996 analysis of this topic, Crepaz-Keay concluded that 'almost all newspapers doubled the frequency of homicides found by the inquiry to have been committed by mentally ill people. This exaggeration includes the Telegraph (17th August 1994, p.1) and the Times (17th August 1994, p.5) broadsheet newspapers. Television drama also represents a disproportionately high amount of violence amongst the mentally disordered. Gerbner *et al.*, (1981) found that 17% of all prime time American television drama included a character who was experiencing mental disorder. Of this group, 73% were portrayed as violent and 23% as homicidal. This stands in contrast to the figures for those characters deemed not to be experiencing mental disorder of 40% and 10% respectively.

Thirdly, the reporting of this inquiry also highlights how a social problem can be singled out as especially threatening when it is no greater a threat than other social problems. The inquiry team considered homicides committed in England and Wales by people who had contact with psychiatric services in the 12 months prior to the killing. Over the 1991-1993 period, some 34 such episodes were recorded. As the Inquiry team's 1996 report observes, this compares with the average of 500 homicide convictions obtained each year in Britain (Steering Committee, 1996). The killing of people by those who may be experiencing mental disorder must be taken seriously and, where possible, amendments made to services in the light of this and similar data which may reduce this figure. However, this approach should also be taken to the hugely greater number of deaths where the perpetrator did not have contact with psychiatric services in the preceding 12 months. The disproportionately greater degree of media coverage for the deaths considered by the Inquiry did not reflect this.

Fourthly, it is often assumed that the risk of violence presented by those experiencing mental disorder is greater than the similar risk posed at other times. Sayce (1995) believes that the myth of growing patient violence has taken a firm hold, despite the unlikelihood of this. The finding that former patients who do not misuse illicit drugs or alcohol have similar rates of violence as do their non-patient neighbours (Steadman *et al.*, 1998) may more accurately reflect the longer term nature of this problem and prompt its proportional consideration as part of a wider social problem.

The key elements of the various analyses of moral panics reflect, to a large extent, the position of those experiencing enduring disorder, and the perception of the risk of violence presented by this group. This is especially evident in the years immediately following the passing of the

*NHS and Community Care Act* (House of Commons, 1990), where the moral panic was fuelled by some spectacular failures in community care.
Evidence for Cohen's (1972) analysis of moral panic in relation to 'serious mental illness' is available in both the news and entertainment media and, to some extent, in the literature of mental health professionals. Here examples of language that is, at best, immoderate for journal publications can be found that parallel the unsubstantiated and over generalised tones of their tabloid and broadsheet counterparts.

1.  The first stage here determines that someone or thing must be defined as a threat to society's values or interests. Violence and murder will be seen by most as fulfilling these threat criteria. The sensationalist reporting of homicides committed by those experiencing serious mental disorder contributes to the definition of these acts as a significant threat to society's values and interests. The compulsory community supervision of individuals thought to present such a risk may be seen to reflect moral panic (Holloway, 1996). The media's narrowing of the public image of 'serious mental illness' has been implicated in the development of moral panic by McRobbie and Thornton (1995).

2.  This narrowed perspective parallels Cohen's (1972) second key element of moral panic, that the threat must be depicted in an easily recognisable form by the media. The application by the media of a rather limited glossary of mental health terms to behaviours which range from that which is slightly less than mainstream to that which is evident of mental disorder, contributes to this sense of moral panic.

3.  Cohen (1972) describes the requirement of tabloid build-up of public concern as his third key element, and this may be seen to have been variable in the serious mental illness debate over the past decade. Early examples of poor community mental health care reasonably sparked public concerns for this group's experience of community resettlement which was marked, in many instances, by indecent haste. Low points here include the killing of Jonathan Zito and Ben Silcock's invasion of the lion's den at London Zoo in 1992 (Appendix 1).

4.  Most would agree that these events contributed to the setting up of the Department of Health's internal working party on compulsory community care. Cohen (1972) describes this response from authorities and opinion makers as the fourth stage in his model. The introduction of supervision registers in 1994 and some of the conclusions of the

1994 *Mental Health Nursing Review* (DoH, 1994a) seem also to be, in part, a response to the highly publicised Zito killing.

5. The extent to which the moral panic associated with those experiencing enduring disorder, and the risk of violence posed by them, has receded seems debatable. Cohen (1972) observed that the panic often does recede, or it results in a social change occurring. In the case of those with enduring disorder the panic has receded, and social and professional change has taken place. Psychiatric services have, since the early nineties, increasingly focused their attention on this client group (DoH, 1994a). Moral panic has driven policy toward increasing control of the 'mentally ill' and this has been based on the perception that violence by mentally ill people is increasing and that community care policies are responsible for a rise in violent crime in Britain (Holloway, 1996).

Moral panic in relation to those experiencing enduring disorder, and the level of violence risk presented by them, has been evidenced at a variety of points across the 1990s in Britain. As a quote from Cohen (1972, p. 67) argues, this has:

> ...become defined as a threat to societal values and interests; its nature is presented in a stylised and stereotyped fashion by the mass media; the moral barricades are manned by editors, politicians and other right thinking people; socially accredited experts pronounce their diagnosis and solutions; ways of coping are evolved (more often) resorted to.

In this instance of moral panic, its legacy has been a significant one. The reorientation of mental health policy and services to those experiencing enduring disorder has changed society's conception of those thought to be the legitimate recipients of psychiatric and mental health care. This reorientation of services may be viewed as less than a coincidental result of an orchestrated public outcry on community care.

In Jenkins' (1992) study of moral panic, he found in each instance a number of influential individuals with either a set of interests, or a political agenda. That this moral panic involves crime, lends it to an understanding from the 'elite engineered' perspective (Chambliss and Mankoff, 1976). Here the suppression of crime may be seen to enable the ruling stratum to 'maintain its privileged position'. This model may be extended to the professional discourse on the topic, where the targeting of enduring disorder may be seen as enabling psychiatry to strengthen its grip on mental health care. This would contribute to psychiatry's maintenance of its privileged social and professional status in a post community care era. Medical domination of other mental health professionals is strengthened here where those labelled as 'seriously mentally ill' frequently benefit from psychotropic medication. That the use of these drugs is derived from medical knowledge and research further undermines the autonomy of non-medical mental health workers and contributes to medical dominance (Friedson, 1974). The unequal status of non-medical mental health care workers in comparison to their medical colleagues, and the usual requirement that these workers' contribution to care is requested by the medical practitioner who makes the diagnosis and is involved in the treatment, also contributes to medical domination (*ibid*). These factors have long been understood, and the targeting of a client group often deemed to be ill and frequently requiring in-patient initial assessment and treatment, further reinforces the imbalance in power between the professionals.

Community care may have threatened, for a short while, to de-stabilise this control, with a shift in emphasis from the medical model to a wellness model (Armentrout, 1993) increasingly adopted by mental health nurses and other professions allied to medicine. Certainly, the concept of empowerment, embraced by the World Health Organisation in its *Ottawa Charter* on health promotion (WHO, 1986) is inconsistent with the medical model, where individuals are urged to take control of their health (Table 3.2). It is particularly relevant to mental health promotion, where compelling arguments exist for a range of measures from the empowerment of consumers, to the establishment of consumer controlled services. Empowerment's three general attributes, self-determination, social engagement and a sense of personal competence (Dickerson, 1998), compete directly with the assumptions of the medical model.

Self-esteem is at the heart of empowerment, where it is associated with a positive attitude about oneself and a feeling of self worth (Rosenberg, 1965). As a product of social feedback and self-appraisal, empowerment may be affected by personal experience and therapeutic interventions (Bednar and Peterson, 1995). However, the concept of empowerment lacks sufficient empirical grounding to be considered an independent construct (Dickerson, 1998), and this may have contributed to the wellness model's lack of credibility within the prevailing scientific paradigm which dominates mental health research.

## Table 3.2  Wellness critique of the medical model

- Problem orientation - Medical education and experience deal primarily with illness and weaknesses to the exclusion of patient strengths and reactions to life events and environment.

- Focus on what is wrong - This often negative and pessimistic approach reinforces the concept of waiting until something happens before making lifestyle changes.

- Focus on patient parts - This often leads to labelling and the marginalisation of the mind and spirit's contribution to wellness.

- Prevention of disease - This maybe relevant if the medical model assumptions are accepted, if it excludes the promotion of health.

- Treatment of symptoms - This often results in the causes of the problem being overlooked. The basic human needs of those experiencing enduring problems are often overlooked by mental health professionals, where higher priority is often given to the 'symptoms' of 'serious mental illness'.

- Treatments are artificial - The risk and treatment of iatrogenic conditions are frequently ill considered. The assessment of extra pyramidal symptoms are seldom assessed systematically. Also, the involvement of patients and their carers in reaching informed decisions about the use of powerful psychotropics is seldom realised.

- Diet as a treatment - The medical focus has been on the propensity of some foods to exacerbate problems, rather than their potential to promote wellness. One need look no further than the typical psychiatric hospital menu for evidence that this is frequently the case! The use of complementary approaches in psychiatry in Britain has been slow to become established despite evidence of their efficacy, for example, the use of St. John's Wort in treating depression.

- Causes of disease are external - People are seen as passive victims rather than having the potential to make healthy lifestyle changes. Personal competence has traditionally been considered an irrelevance, where the locus of control in relation to health behaviours was assumed to be completely independent of the hypothesised pathological agent. The development of psychological approaches to enduring disorder over the last decade is, to some degree, a reaction to this position. Here, the client is assumed to be able to exert some control over the processing of information with the effect that the residual positive features of enduring disorder may be better understood and controlled.

- External control - Clients are expected to submit powerlessly to prescribed treatments and relinquish notions of self-determination. Those experiencing enduring disorder have traditionally been expected to give up control of their lives to health professionals, and this contributes to the promotion of dependency, frequently seen in those who have acquired the 'institutionalised' label.

- Fear as a motivator - Fear is frequently used to maintain compliance to a regime of care, or a prescription, with which the client may disagree. This may be more prevalent in the one-to-one consultation. This manipulation may be subtle and more evident where the client is vulnerable through poor social integration.

- Aspiritual - There is no spiritual component to the medical model, and the acceptance of this effectively blocks off an important avenue of comfort and support to the many who would benefit from the acknowledgement and development of this aspect of human existence.

- Quality of life - The medical model promotes the use of extreme measures to maintain life often with little regard for the quality of it.

*Source:* Adapted from Armentrout, (1993).

This competition, posed by the wellness model, may be seen as a threat to psychiatry that has been slow to embrace the consumers' agenda. The features of the wellness model are highlighted in Table 3.2 via the critique of the medical model. Unfortunately, many of these criticisms are valid today, despite the many years of wider consumer empowerment enjoyed in Britain.

The shoring up of the medical model by moral panic may also stabilise the socio-economic status of the medical profession in relation to other mental health care workers, who tend to enjoy a lower level of social status and significantly lower levels of remuneration. The media's coverage of 'serious mental illness' and violence may exemplify the media's tendency to simply reflect the concerns of the powerful in society and, thereby, support the re-establishment of a social order that places the medical profession firmly at the top of the mental health hierarchy.

Other powerful groups would, of course, support this structure of dominance, and it is from the middle portion of this hierarchy that moral panics enjoy their strongest support (Goode and Ben-Yehuda, 1994). Interestingly one of the observations that these authors make is the tendency for the moral panic supporters to influence a variety of social factors which includes the call for new educational curricula. This has been evident in mental health care, where several organisations have campaigned for curricula to reflect core skills in mental health care which are of most direct relevance to those labelled 'seriously mentally ill', for example, the Institute of Psychiatry. Certainly, the structural tendency for this moral panic, caused by the community mental health care failures of the late 1980s and early 1990s, to happily harmonise with the prioritisation of resources via the restriction, or targeting of services, to people experiencing enduring disorder, will be seen by most observers as more than coincidental. The exaggeration of the risk of violence posed by this group must be seen as a major contributory factor in the relative ease with which the government have 'pulled-off' this targeting exercise, with little opposition to the concomitant marginalisation of those experiencing mental disorders not deemed to be 'serious'.

## Conclusion

That the news and entertainment media's coverage of mental health issues in the early to mid 1990s constituted a moral panic seems now beyond doubt. Much less clarity surrounds the role of the key stakeholders - mental health professionals, government, carer and consumer groups and the public - in initiating and maintaining this state of affairs, let alone their motivation and gains deriving from it. It can be concluded that this moral panic most probably strengthened the hand of psychiatry in the mental health arena, and this will be perceived as a regrettable step backwards by the majority of mental health workers. The modernist position of psychiatry is further maintained by this moral panic, despite the move to post modernity by other major institutions, where the consumers' view of reality is considered central to their interface and satisfaction with the services offered. The wellness perspective is some way off in British psychiatry, and its acceptance has not been hastened by this moral panic. It has certainly supported the targeting of the 'seriously mentally ill', despite the ethical anomalies arising from the marginalisation of those deemed to be less of a priority. Only the naïve would believe the occurrence of this, at a time when prioritisation and rationing are at the fore front of policy thinking, to be a coincidence. It is also clear that this panic was triggered by some very real and regrettable community care calamities, if the response to these was disproportionate in the extreme. In addition, there may be a real increased risk of violence posed by this group which mental health workers may find unpalatable. The assessment of this risk will continue to be crucial to effective community care for this group, albeit that much research is left yet to be done in this area.

## References

American Psychiatric Association (APA)   (1994), *Diagnostic and Statistical Manual of Mental Disorders*, American Psychiatric Association, Washington.

Armentrout, G. (1993), 'A Comparison of the Medical Model and the Wellness Model: The Importance of Knowing the Difference', *Holistic Nursing Practice*, vol. 7 no. 4, pp. 57-62.

Audit Commission (1986), *Making a Reality of Community Care*, Audit Commission, London.

Barker, P.J., Keady, J., Croom, S., Stevenson, C, Adams, T. and Reynolds, W. (1998), 'The Concept of Serious Mental Illness: Modern Myths and Grim Realities', *Journal of Psychiatric and Mental Health Nursing*, vol. 5, pp. 247-54.

Bednar, R.L. and Peterson, S.R. (1995), *Self-Esteem: Paradoxes and Innovations in Clinical Theory and Practice*, American Psychological Association, Washington.

Berger, P.L. and Luckman, T. (1968), *The Social Construction of Reality*, Doubleday, New York.

Bloom, J. (1989), 'The Character of Danger in Psychiatric Practice: Are the Mentally Ill Dangerous?', *Bulletin of the American Academy of Psychiatry and the Law*, vol. 17, pp. 241-54.

Bowers, L. (1997), 'CPN Caseloads and the 'Worried Well': Misspent Time or Vital Work?', *Journal of Advanced Nursing*, vol. 26, pp. 930-6.

Brennan, C. (1995), 'Beyond Theory and Practice: A Postmodern Perspective', *Counseling and Values*, vol. 39, January, pp. 99-107.

Cardinal, M. (1996), 'The Words To Say It', in, S. Dunn, B. Morrison, and M. Roberts, *Mind Readings: Writers' Journeys Through Mental States*, Minerva, London.

Chambliss, W. and Mankoff, M. (eds) (1976), *Whose Law? What Order?*, Wiley, New York. Cited in, Thomson, K. (1998), *Op Cit.*

Cohen, S. (1972), *Folk Devils and Moral Panics: The Creation of the Mods and Rockers*, MacGibbon and Kee, London.

Confidential Inquiry into Homicides and Suicides by Mentally Ill People (1994), *Preliminary Report on Homicide*, Department of Health, London.

Crepaz-Keay, D. (1996), 'A Sense of Perspective: the Media and the Boyd Inquiry, in Philo, G. (1996), *Op Cit.*

Denzin, N. J. (1991), *Images of Postmodern Society*, Sage, Newbury Park, California.

Department of Health (1990), *Care Programme Approach for People with a Mental Illness Referred to the Specialist Psychiatric Services*, HC(90)23/LASSL(90)11, Department of Health, London.

Department of Health (1993), 'Legal Powers on the Care of Mentally Ill People in the Community', *Report of the Internal Review*, Department of Health, London.

Department of Health (1994a), *Working in Partnership; Report of the Mental Health Nursing Review Team*, HMSO, London.

Department of Health (1994b), Introduction of Supervision Registers for Mentally Ill People from 1 April 1994, (HSG(94)5), Department of Health, London.

Department of Health and Social Security Memorandum 1983), *Mental Health Act*, HMSO, London.

Deutsch, A. (1949), The Mentally Ill in America: A History of Their Care and Treatment from Colonial Times (2$^{nd}$ ed.), Columbia University Press, New York. Cited in, Monahan, J. (1992), *Op Cit.*

Dickerson, F.B. (1998), 'Strategies that Foster Empowerment', *Cognitive and Behavioural Practice*, vol. 5, no. 2, pp. 255-75.

Dreyfus, H. and Dreyfus, S. (1986), *Mind Over Machine*, The Free Press, New York.

Ennis, B. and Emery, R. (1978), *The Rights of Mental Patients – An American Civil Liberties Union Handbook*, Avon, New York.

Foucault, M. (1972), *The Archaeology of Knowledge,* Tavistock, London.

Friedson, E. (1974), 'Dominant Professions Bureaucracy and Client Services', in, Y. Hassenfeld and R.A. English (eds.), *Human Service Organizations*, University of Michigan Press, Ann Arbor, Michigan.

Gerbner, G., Gross, L., Morgan, M. and Signorielli, N. (1981), 'Health and Medicine on Television', *The New England Journal of Medicine*, vol. 305, pp. 901-4.

Goode, E. and Ben-Yehuda (1994), *Moral Panics: The Social Construction of Deviance*, Blackwell, Oxford and Cambridge, Massachusetts.

Gournay, K. (1994), 'Redirecting the Emphasis to Serious Mental Illness', *Nursing Times*, vol. 90, no. 25, pp. 40-1.

Holloway, F. (1996), 'Community Psychiatric Care: From Libertarianism to Coercion. Moral Panic and Mental Health Policy in Britain', *Health Care Analysis*, vol. 4, no. 3, pp. 235-43.

Horkheimer, M. (1972), *Critical Theory*, Seabury, New York.

Jenkins, P (1992), *Intimate Enemies: Moral Panics in Contemporary Great Britain*, Aldine de Gruyter, New York.

House of Commons (1983), *The Mental Health Act*, HMSO, London.

House of Commons (1985), *The Second Report of the Social Services Committee,* HMSO, London.
House of Commons (1990), *NHS and Community Care Act,* HMSO, London.
Kingdon, D. and Jenkins, R. (1996), 'Adult Mental Health Policy', in G. Thornicroft and G. Strathdee, *Commissioning Mental Health Services,* Gaskell, London.
Lacan, J. (1977), Ecrits, W.W. Norton, New York. Cited in, Murphy, J. (1989), 'Clinical Intervention in the Postmodern World', *International Journal of Adolescence and Youth,* vol. 2, no. 1, pp. 61-9.
Lloytard, J.F. (1984), *The Postmodern Condition: A Report on Knowledge,* University of Minnesota Press, Minneapolis.
Matarazzo, W. (1986), *Iconology: Image, Text, Ideology.* University of Chicago Press, Chicago.
McFadyen, J.A. and Farrington, A. (1996), 'The Failure of Community Care for the Severely Mentally Ill', *British Journal of Nursing,* vol. 5, no. 15, pp. 920-8.
McRobbie, A. and Thornton, S.L. (1995), 'Rethinking Moral Panic for Multi-Mediated Social Worlds', *British Journal of Sociology,* vol. 46, no. 4, pp.559-74.
Mitchell, J.W.T. (1986), *Iconology,* University of Chicago Press, Chicago.
Monahan, J. (1992), 'Mental Disorder and Violent Behaviour: Perceptions and Evidence', *American Psychologist,* April, pp. 511-21.
Monahan, J. and Steadman, H. (1983), Crime and Mental Disorder: an Epidemiological Approach, in, .N. Morris and M. Tonry (eds.), *Crime and Justice: An Annual Review of Research,* University of Chicago Press, Chicago.
Murphy, J. (1976), 'Psychiatric Labelling in Cross-cultural Perspective', *Science,* vol. 191, pp. 1019-28.
Murphy, J. (1989), 'Clinical Intervention in the Postmodern World', *International Journal of Adolescence and Youth,* vol. 2. no. 1, pp. 61-9.
Neuchterlein, K. and Dawson, M. (1984), 'A Heuristic Vulnerability-Stress Model of Schizophrenia Episodes', *Schizophrenia Bulletin,* vol. 10, pp. 300-12.
Pardeck, J.T. and Murphy, J.W. (1993), 'Postmodernism and Clinical Practice: A Critical Analysis of the Disease Model', *Psychological Reports,* vol. 72, pp. 1187-94.
Pescosolido, B. A., Monahan, J., Link, B.G., Stueve, A. and Kikuzawa, S. (1999), 'The Public's View of the Competence, Dangerousness, and Need for Legal Coercion of Persons With Mental Health Problems', *American Journal of Public Health,* vol. 89, no. 9, pp. 1339-45.
Philo, G. (Ed.) (1996), *Media and Mental Distress,* Longman, London.
Ritchie, J.H., Dick, D. and Lingham, R. (1994), *The Report of the Inquiry into the Care and Treatment of Christopher Clunis,* HMSO, London.
Robertson, G. (1988), 'Arrest Patterns Among Mentally Disordered Offenders', *British Journal of Psychiatry,* vol. 153, pp. 313-16.
Rosen, G. (1968), *Madness in Society: Chapters in the Historical Sociology of Mental Illness,* University of Chicago Press, Chicago.

Rosenberg, M. (1965), 'Society and the Adolescent Self-Image', Princeton University Press, Princeton. Cited in, F.B. Dickerson (1998), *Op Cit.*

Royal College of Psychiatrists (1993), *Community Supervision Orders*, Royal College of Psychiatrists, London.

Sayce, L. (1995), Response to Violence: 'A Framework for Fair Treatment', in, J. Crichton (Ed.), *Psychiatric Patient Violence, Risk and Response*, Duckworth, London.

Schon, D. (1991), *The Reflective Practitioner 2nd edition*, Josey Bass, San Francisco.

Spokes, J. (Chairman) (1988), *Report of the Committee of Inquiry into the Care and Aftercare of Sharon Campbell*, HMSO, London.

Steadman, H.J., Mulvey, E.P. and Monahan, J., Clark Robbins, P., Appelbaum, P.S., Grisso, T., Roth, L.H. and Silver, E. (1998), 'Violence by People Discharged From Acute Psychiatric Inpatient Facilities and by Others in the Same Neighborhoods', *Archives of General Psychiatry*, vol. 55, pp. 393-401.

Steering Committee of the Confidential Enquiry into Homicides and Suicides by Mentally Ill People (1996), *Report of the Confidential Enquiry into Homicides and Suicides by Mentally Ill People,* Royal College of Psychiatrists, London.

Thomson, J.B. (1984), Studies in the Theory of Ideology, University of California Press, Berkeley. Cited in, J.T. Pardeck and J.W. Murphy (1993), *Op Cit.*

Thomson, K. (1998), *Moral Panics*, Routledge, London.

Waddington, P.A.J. (1986), 'Mugging as a Moral Panic: A Question of Proportion', *British Journal of Sociology*, vol. 37, no. 2, pp. 245-59.

Wessely, S. and Taylor, P. (1991), 'Madness and Crime: Criminology vs. Psychiatry', *Criminal Behaviour and Mental Health*, vol. 1, pp.193-228.

Westermeyer, J. and Kroll, J. (1978), 'Violence and Mental Illness in a Peasant Society: Characteristics of Violent Behaviours and 'Folk' Use of Restraints', *British Journal of Psychiatry*, vol. 133, pp. 529-41.

White, D.R. and Hellerich, G. (1992), 'Postmodern Reflections on Modern Psychiatry: The Diagnostic and Statistical Manual of Mental Disorders', *The Humanistic Psychologist*, vol. 20, no. 1, pp. 75-91.

World Health Organization (WHO) (1986), *Ottawa Charter for Health Promotion*, World Health Organization, Ottawa.

World Health Organization (1992), *The ICD-10 Classification of Mental and Behavioural Disorders: Clinical Descriptions and Diagnostic Guidelines*, World Health Organization, Geneva.

Young, J. (1971), The role of the police as amplifiers of deviance, negotiators of drug control as seen in Notting Hill. In, S. Cohen (Ed.) *Images of Deviance*, Penguin, Harmondsworth.

## Appendix 1: Chronological account of significant events linking mental disorder with violence

1985 - The Social Services Select Committee of the House of Commons (House of Commons, 1985) expressed concern about community care and have subsequently been many times quoted as claiming that 'any fool can close a mental hospital: it takes time and effort to do it properly and compassionately'.

1986 - The Audit Commission (1986) expressed concern about community care in its publication *Making a Reality of Community Care.*

1988 - *Report of the Committee of Inquiry into the Care and Aftecare of Sharon Campbell.* Sharon Campbell experienced enduring mental disorder and killed social worker Isobel Schwarz. The report emphasised the importance of interprofessional collaboration, systematic assessment and aftercare (Spokes, 1988; Kingdon and Jenkins, 1996).

1990 – Government publish its proposal for the introduction of the care programme approach for those who had been referred to the specialist psychiatric services (DoH, 1990).

1991, April - Care programme approach introduced in all district health authorities.

1992 - The Department of Health establish its *Confidential Enquiry into Homicides and Suicides by Mentally Ill People.* This made recommendations, in 1994 (Confidential Enquiry, 1994), for best practice and included discussion on avoidable causes of death.

1992 - Christopher Clunis stabbed Jonathan Zito (Ritchie *et al.,* 1994). Ben Silcock climbed into the lions' den at London zoo and footage of this was shown on national television news.

1993 - The Royal College of Psychiatrists recommended the introduction of compulsory supervision orders (Royal College of Psychiatrists, 1993). This measure was designed to permit the speedy recall of patients who had been previously compulsorily detained under the M*ental Health Act* (House of Commons, 1983) in a psychiatric hospital if they refused to undergo further treatment.

1993 - The Department of Health internal working party on compulsory community care was established.

1993, August - The working party recommended that supervised discharge should be introduced.

1994, February - The Ritchie report on the killing of Jonathan Zito highlighted many examples of the inadequacies in the care of Christopher Clunis.

1994, April - Supervision registers were introduced to 'ensure that SMI people who are at greatest need receive the services they require' (DoH, 1994b).

1994 - The Department of Health mental health nursing review estimated that 80% of people diagnosed as having schizophrenia were not receiving input from a community psychiatric nurse (DoH, 1994a).

# PART 2
# PERSPECTIVES ON
# TARGETING

# 4 A Psychiatrist's Perspective.
IAN DAVIDSON

## Introduction

This chapter explores the meaning of 'targeting' and the issues surrounding it from the perspective of a clinical psychiatrist. The author is a Consultant Psychiatrist with 19 years of practice, 12 of which have been spent as a Consultant in an inner city catchment area, and involved academic and educational roles, as well as management roles such as Clinical Director. The views expressed in this chapter reflect some of the experiences and observations gained during that career. The chapter begins by 'unpacking' the notion of targeting in mental health services, highlighting aspects of targeting which set the agenda for clinical practice. Next, some of the advantages and disadvantages of targeting are reviewed. Then, the future of targeting is explored in relation to national policy developments and initiatives. Throughout the chapter, relevant examples are included to illustrate particular issues. The chapter is concluded with a brief discussion of the key principles involved in targeting.

## What Does 'Targeting' Mean in Relation to Clinical Mental Health?

In my opinion this is the key question. I believe that it can be subdivided into three components:

- targeting of what?
- targeting by whom and/or what?
- targeting for what?

### Targeting of What?

At whom, or what, is the targeting aimed? The *Health of the Nation Key Area Handbook for Mental Illness* (DoH, 1993) identified two sets of targets for mental illness. One set dealt with reducing suicide rates. The other was intended to '...improve significantly the health and social functioning of mentally ill people'. These are important aims and they define the target group as being mainly those people with some form of mental illness. Depending on definitions, this could be between 15% and 20% of the adult population in any given week. In *Building Bridges,* the secondary specialist mental health services in the NHS in the U.K. were directed to '...target their resources first and foremost on severely mentally ill people' (DoH, 1995). Clearly, 'serious mental illness' (SMI) has been identified as a priority. Whilst the term 'severe or enduring mental illness' (SEMI) is sometimes used inter-changeably with the term SMI, they are not identical. Nevertheless, there is reasonable agreement about the core type of problems that fulfill this description, although there is much less agreement about the boundaries. 'Severe' and 'enduring' are both relative terms, and are thus different from different perspectives. However, the reality is that multiple targeting is expected, even within mental illness services. Examples include targeting of the homeless, mentally disordered offenders, people from ethnic communities, children and adolescents, women, the young, the old, the isolated, those perceived as being at risk, and so on.

## Targeting by Whom and/or What?

Even when a definite target group is identified, competing demands still exist. The problem for a clinical team is what proportion of their resources should be allocated to the target group? In a few very specialised services with a very tightly defined target group, this may involve the whole team. In primary and secondary care teams, multiple expectations and targets are the norm. Often the demands of different, competing needs exceed the total team resource. Targeting then becomes a matter of prioritising on a day-to-day basis, trying to balance maximum benefit against least harm. It is, therefore, crucial for a team to have an accurate knowledge of local resources, and to know how to deploy those resources to best effect.

*Local Services for People with Mental Health Problems* (DoH, 1996) made it clear that 90% of mental health problems were expected to be dealt with at the primary care level. This implied that only about 10% of the most severe cases should have access to specialist services. Rising demand on primary care services can lead to increased pressure on secondary services, particularly if the 10% threshold is exceeded.

*Targeting for What?*

What is the desired outcome? This is very subjective. No intervention is free of consequences. Two current jargon terms illustrate this issue. Promoting positive health by increasing autonomy involves risk-taking. Harm reduction involves trying to reduce risk. They are not mutually exclusive, but it is easy to see that they can often be in conflict. A good outcome also depends on perspective. Locking someone into lifelong solitary confinement probably reduces the risk of him or her hurting another person. Again, it is easy to see that from a range of other perspectives this could be a very bad outcome. Ill-defined outcomes are a common reason why expectations exceed ability to deliver. Given that a gain to one group, from some form of targeting, usually results in a loss to another group, clear outcomes and transparent decision making are essential in order to reduce the risk of conflict.

A series of government papers have tried to address this issue. The Care Programme Approach (CPA) introduced in 1991 (DoH, 1990) requires each person in contact with any specialist mental health professional to have a care plan and a named key worker. This is good, but even where the paperwork is completed, doubts remain about the value of the exercise. This is because it can be seen as a form-filling exercise rather than a dynamic care plan with clear objectives and strategies. The philosophy is correct and, if used sensibly, it can enhance targeting of individual needs.

*Modernising Mental Health Services* (DoH, 1998) sets out current government policy for England and Wales. This defines the major principles to underpin NHS spending and investment in mental health and, thereby, sketches in the background against which targeting initiatives must be developed and evaluated. The key objectives are to deliver 'safe, sound and supportive' mental health services. In principle, these are to be applauded. The reality is that the true targeting debates can only start once the implementation groups for the national service framework (NSF) become operational. The evidence is that the government is trying to be more explicit about the need to balance expectations against the allocated resources whilst, at the same time, trying to maximise the benefits gained from the resources. This promotes a culture in which rational discussion of targeting can take place. This is welcome and, if followed through, should improve services and help to address the current major recruitment and retention problems that exists for skilled staff in adult mental illness services in England and Wales.

## Advantages of Targeting

Given the reality of finite resources, it is essential that they be put to greatest use. The advantages of targeting address this point, and include:

- effectiveness;
- efficiency;
- efficacy; and,
- goal-setting.

### *Effectiveness*

'Effective' refers to the extent to which stated goals are achieved. The increasing emphasis on evidence-based medicine (Sackett *et al.*, 1997) is leading to clearer knowledge of what will produce positive results. Examples of this process are contained in the Cochrane database. Preferentially purchasing effective, evidence-based approaches is an example of good targeting. The National Institute for Clinical Excellence (NICE) should also aid this process by the development of appropriate guidelines. The current reality is that the amount of information available is overwhelming in volume, but of very uneven quality. The increasing emphasis on teaching critical appraisal skills at undergraduate and postgraduate levels is, therefore, essential. Only by the use of those skills can the best evidence be determined.

### *Efficiency*

'Efficient' means that greatest effect is achieved for least input. The proper use of resources requires that, where two or more approaches achieve similar effect, then the least costly should be chosen. This again is good targeting. An example of using this sort of approach at a local level is provided by the 'Home Support Treatment' initiative (HoST) in Liverpool. This initiative was funded through Liverpool Health Authority to try to tackle the problems of bed occupancy running at over 100%. The aim was to identify people with SMI at risk of hospitalisation, and to try to reduce this risk by enhancing their home treatment. Clear protocols were devised. The initial target group included people who had a history of repeated and/or lengthy admissions in the previous two years. The use of protocols and outcome measures clearly showed that spreading the resource across the whole target group would not be efficient, as the resource would be spread too thinly to be effective. Analysis of the data showed that the most efficient use of the service required targeting the people who were on level 3 CPA, despite full input from standard services (Davidson and Cowley, 1998).

*Efficacy*

'Efficacy' refers to producing the desired effect. An effective treatment may be efficient, but may not be the most efficacious due to too many unwanted effects. This reality is commonly acknowledged in relation to pharmacological therapies, i.e., where the choice between two or more equally effective treatments is determined by the side effect profile.

*Goal-Setting*

Another advantage of targeting in mental health concerns accuracy in identifying people at increased risk. At the level of individual teams, assigning cases to the CPA levels 1, 2 or 3 indicated priorities for resources within the team at that time (DoH, 1990, now superseded by DoH, 1999a). This sort of targeting is used to increase the opportunity for high-risk individuals or groups to get the best help within available resources. Another approach is to identify specific protected resources for certain groups. Examples of this approach include specialised teams for the homeless, assertive outreach teams and screening programmes. In all of these cases, it should be noted that identifying higher risk cases without shifting resources is not targeting. It must also be remembered that shifting resources means reducing resources elsewhere, and the effects of this on the population must be taken into account. Once resources have moved from one service to another, they can be very hard to transfer back! The perception of general, adult psychiatrists is that a greater proportion of resources has shifted to specialised services than have patients.

## Disadvantages of Targeting

The disadvantages of targeting include:

- exclusion;
- disillusionment;
- over-inclusion;
- misdirection;
- fashion;
- elitism; and,
- stigma.

### *Exclusion*

The most obvious disadvantage of targeting is exclusion. Targeting of a specific resource to an individual, or group of people, inevitably means that others can not have it. This is only likely to create problems if demand for that particular resource exceeds supply, or if the wrong people are excluded. The total demand for specialist mental health services from the NHS currently exceeds supply. The national policy is that people with SMI should have priority. This means that many people with mild to moderate mental illnesses have little or no priority. A risk of targeting would be to simply ignore this issue, i.e., if you are not in a target group, you have no relevance. Targeting one group should not lead to the assumption that the excluded have no needs, and this is likely to remain a contentious issue. The above is at least planned exclusion, and in a transparent decision-making process the rationale is open to challenge and debate.

A more insidious problem is non-explicit exclusion. Approaches that are based upon doing the best for the person presenting at that time (e.g., the GMC guidance *Duties of a Doctor*) are essentially targeting by access. Taken literally, and given finite resources, this approach has major flaws. Treating the first patient in clinic in the best possible way means that less is available for the second, and so on. This means that place in the queue determines quality of care. In reality no service can operate safely or fairly in that manner, and some attempt has to be made to share out resources rationally. Even so, the inherent bias of doing the best for the person in front of you at that time places a great premium on getting access. Targeting which does not take account of access issues will inevitably increase this bias. Access can involve relatively straightforward issues such as distance and timing, but in mental health issues like waiting time, the use of pre-appointment questionnaires, stigma, ethnicity and/or language factors may also distort free access.

An accidental by-product of targeting can be deceit. This is especially likely where the gap in provision between the target group and the excluded group is very large. Most clinicians are aware of cases where patients and/or the referring agency alter details to enable access to a particular service.

## *Disillusionment*

Targeting that is vague can lead to demand exceeding supply. In the worst scenario this can lead to no-one getting an acceptable service. In general adult psychiatry this problem has contributed significantly to poor job satisfaction, poor recruitment and poor retention of skilled staff of all disciplines. In some parts of the country, this has led to services only being available through a series of locums. It is a daily dilemma in adult psychiatry as to whether to give person A the best service, or to reduce that service so that persons B and C get some service. This 'robbing Peter to pay Paul' is common in all walks of life, but it creates great anxiety when it is perceived that any subsequent inquiries only focus on whether A got the best service, regardless of other issues. These issues are acknowledged in *Modernising Mental Health Services* (DoH, 1998) under 'failures of the past'. This has been where the GMC type of guidance has been essential to ensure that at least some people got an adequate service. It is to be hoped that clear targeting and adequate resourcing to meet the chosen targets will ensure that all those eligible for the service get an adequate service.

## *Over-Inclusion*

Over-inclusion is another risk of targeting. In this case, a scarce resource may be spread too thinly by vague inclusion criteria. An example of this was the inclusion of a patient in 'Compliance Therapy' when he was fully compliant and had different needs. Most of these over-inclusions do no direct harm, but they waste resources that could be better used.

## *Misdirection*

Targeting can also be misdirected. In the HoST example referred to earlier (Davidson and Cowley, 1998), the initial target was determined by historic bed usage. This was a reasonable place to start, but this group included people whose care plans had already been altered to successfully improve their treatment. Giving additional input to these people would have been in line with the protocol, but would have produced no significant benefit at high cost. We also identified that some people on CPA level 3 were at risk, but did not qualify on historic data, despite being likely to benefit from the service. In this case, the protocol was amended successfully. In many instances such ongoing review and revision does not take place. This can result in targeting resources at a fixed problem when the world has moved on to other issues.

*Fashion*

One of the major reasons for misdirected targeting is 'fashion'. Someone has heard of a new initiative in another place, and thinks local services should adopt this approach. This is an important way of stopping services becoming insular and outmoded if it is used to stimulate debate about the needs and aims of local services. However, it can lead to serious misdirection, if services from elsewhere are simply adopted without first clearly identifying risks and benefits to local services overall. This is particularly a risk where the proposed targeting change is driven by vested interests and special pleading. Such activities are vital to promoting new approaches, but enthusiasm can not be a substitute for taking an overall view of the impact on needs and services. Such vested interests include pharmacological companies, professional groups, patient groups, politicians and many more.

*Elitism*

Elitism can have harmful aspects in relation to targeting. It can lead to arrogance and a "closed shop" mentality. It can also lead to burnout, if expectations exceed ability to deliver. This is a particular risk where services have been set up by dynamic, charismatic leaders, who then move on after a relatively short time. In mental health, services need time to mature, and real outcomes can take years to become apparent, whether for good or bad. Expectations must also take account of the 'population attributable fraction'. In essence, this means that even if the planned intervention can totally eliminate the targeted problem, how much will it reduce the population health risk. Elitism, therefore, appears as both a potential advantage and disadvantage. Recognition of services advancing good practice, Beacon services, encourages them and other services. Failure to review and evaluate can lead to elite services gaining resources out of proportion to rational targeting for the particular place and time.

*Stigma*

'Target' as a word also has negative connotations. Some people with serious mental health problems see targeting as being directed at them, rather than to help them. The reality of the stigma attached to mental health problems cannot be ignored. This is true both at the general level of British society, and also at many local and sub-cultural levels. Stigma is a complex area, and cannot be simply summarised here. In the context of the reality and perception of stigma, society must be careful that targeting does not get misused as a euphemism for dehumanising people with mentally illness, and disregarding their rights and responsibilities. This leads back to the earlier discussion of targeting for what? The current debates on what should replace the 'Care in the Community' approach, and the debate over revision of the *Mental Health Act* (House of Commons, 1983) reflect unease about the balance between individual rights, duties to society, and the duties of society to the individual. The outcome of these debates is going to have a large impact on the direction of targeting in serious mental illness in the U.K. in the next decade.

**The Future**

The following selection highlights those changes that I believe offer the best opportunities to enhance rational targeting in the future:

- clinical governance;
- information systems;
- critical appraisal;
- CHIMP;
- primary care commissioning;
- modernizing the care programme approach  (DOH, 1999a);
- national service framework for mental health (DOH, 1999b); and,
- review of the Mental Health Act (DoH, 1999c).

*Clinical Governance*

Quality is now firmly on the NHS agenda (DoH, 1998), and clinical governance is the chosen system for delivering this objective. The following quotation from Scally and Donaldson (1998) neatly summarises the process:

> Clinical Governance is a system through which NHS organisations are accountable for continuously improving the quality of their services and safeguarding high standards of care by creating an environment in which excellence in clinical care will flourish.

Clinical governance makes quality a key objective for NHS Boards and Chief Executives. Quality is now at least as important as financial propriety. This is very significant. In the past, change was often perceived as being driven by cost saving measures, regardless of quality or other issues. In future, changes will have to address both the financial realities and the potential quality implications for the service.

*Information Systems*

A major concern in recent years has been the use made of information within the NHS. In at least some services, the quasi-market approach led to a somewhat secretive approach to information. At best, this was unhelpful, and it could virtually stifle stakeholder attempts to promote positive change. The recent policy documents all encourage more sharing of information. The NHS collects much information. Some of this is routine, and some is for specific purposes. Clinical audit is one of those purposes. There has been general dissatisfaction (including from the Audit Commission) with the results of clinical audit. Too often it has been a baseline form filling exercise with no proper outcomes. Used properly, including repeated audit cycles, it can improve targeting and outcomes, and help to refine guidelines. *Modernising Mental Health Services* (DoH, 1998) emphasises the need for better availability of information to clinicians and planners. Clinical governance enables use to be made of that information, both at individual level, and by promoting greater sharing of knowledge.

## Critical Appraisal

Greater access to information places greater importance on developing critical appraisal skills at managerial, as well as, clinical levels. If this is not done, middle managers in particular could become threatened and disempowered by clinical staff and other stakeholders generating new solutions. Managers (or clinicians) lacking these skills may be inclined to fall back on the 'never let the facts get in the way of a good story' approach, which has done so much to prevent sensible planning in the past.

## CHIMP

Only time will tell whether the system outlined in *Modernising Mental Health Services* (DoH, 1998) will be properly funded and supported. The Commission for Health Improvement (CHIMP) will act to promote and monitor the changes. Much of the emphasis is correctly placed upon local reviews of service providers, but it also needs to monitor the wider picture to ensure that the new culture has the necessary support to develop fully.

## Primary Care Commissioning

Primary care commissioning offers the prospect of locally relevant targeting, embracing the needs and total resources of local communities. Conversely, the local nature of primary care commissioning also makes it more vulnerable to the types of distortion and misdirection identified earlier under 'disadvantages of targeting'. Individuals and groups with strong ideas can more easily influence targeting for good or bad. It is my belief, that providing there is the development of appropriate skills and access to timely, accurate information, the benefits will outweigh the potential risks. This is a critical area for the NHS, especially the targeting of mental health resources. It is very encouraging that many PCGs have identified mental health improvement as an urgent priority.

The above developments create real opportunities for targeting decisions to be open and subject to evaluation. Targeting, which is based upon up-to-date and locally relevant information, will be more flexible, and should become more effective, efficient and efficacious. Unlike 'Lily the Pink's medicinal compound', it is unlikely to be efficacious in every case, and that is why the quality reviews built into national frameworks, and monitored through clinical governance and CHIMP, are essential. Setting, delivering and monitoring standards can produce improved quality through targeting, with correct training and access to information. The risk is, that without this, it could simply become an exercise in 'safety first' management with rigid protocols regardless of relevance or practicality: a culture of scapegoating and blame, discouraging initiative and with multiple layers of deniability.

## National Service Framework for Mental Health

The NSF sets out seven key standards for improving mental health services to adults of working age in England (DoH, 1999b). At the time of writing this chapter, it was too soon to know how it will be used in practice, but the document supports and highlights many of the points raised in this chapter. The clear themes that run through it include prioritization; giving explicit reasons for changes and indicating the strength/weakness of the underlying research; and, recognizing the importance of targeting. It gives examples of good practice, whilst acknowledging that these will not fit all communities. Review and revision are inherent to the philosophy. There is an acknowledgment that change takes time and costs resources. The ten-year programme is broken down into key milestones. In my experience it is already helping to improve the quality and transparency of planning in mental health and if this can be maintained over the next ten years, then many of the issues and challenges in this chapter will have been successfully addressed.

## Modernising the Care Programme Approach

The joint NHS/SSI document *Effective Care Co-ordination in Mental Health Services* (DoH, 1999a) uses a similar approach to the NSF. It is clearly less evidence-based than the NSF, but is explicit about the underlying assumptions and uses anecdotal examples of good practice to illustrate potential solutions to identified problems. Given the lack of research in much of mental health service delivery, this is probably the best that can be done at present. In my opinion, this is a clinically useful improvement which does address real issues which have arisen since 1991. In particular, chapter 5 (Achieving a Proper Focus) does acknowledge that positive risk taking is an important element of good care. Recognising the need to balance risks should reduce the risk of the 'safety first', defensive planning as discussed above. This would enable good quality care, whilst ensuring that real safety for the patient and public is always built into any care plan, i.e. taking carefully planned risks in the short-term may be essential to reducing longer-term risks.

## Review of the Mental Health Act

The report of the Expert Committee chaired by Professor Genevra Richardson on the review of the *Mental Health Act* (House of Commons, 1983) led to the *Reform of the Mental Health Act 1983 Proposals for Consultation* (DoH, 1999c) published in November 1999. It is clear from this document that the government does not support all the proposals of the Expert Group. At the time of writing this chapter, it was clear that there is major concern amongst many groups and organizations about the changes, and in particular about compulsory treatment in the community. In contrast to the previous two documents, this does not appear to be evidence-based either by research, or even by good quality, anecdotal reports. The desired aim appears to be reducing serious incidents in the community, but all the inquiries seem to me to demonstrate issues of communication and/or access to services (including inpatient facilities) as being crucial in such incidents.

The other area of concern is that the desire to demonstrate review of patient rights has led to a very intensive programme of reviews and appeals. The document suggests that time spent in formal review hearings contributes to planning of patient care. This is palpable nonsense. Appeals and formal external reviews each take up considerable clinical time (from multiple disciplines). This time is over and above care planning, and indeed the adversarial nature of English legal training means that considerable time may be required after appeals to get the care planning back on track. This is not a reason for ignoring the rights of detained patients, but the resource required needs to be explicitly recognized as the time diverted to this has to come from some other part of the clinical activity.

The process of reviewing the *Mental Health Act* (HMSO, 1983) is essential and many of the proposals are likely to gain general support. The reformed Act should support the NSF and revised CPA, and not be isolated from those policies.

**Conclusion**

In the face of finite resources, targeting of some type is inevitable. In my opinion, it follows from the above that targeting will be beneficial if:

- there is an evidence base for the proposed intervention, and for its use in the defined population;
- benefits of the intervention are balanced against other interventions and/or target groups;
- inputs and outcomes are clearly identified, and under continuous review; and,
- the expectations of patients, carers, therapists, purchasers and public are realistic.

The development of outreach services for the homeless with mental health problems in Liverpool illustrates how targeting can lead to enhanced services using the above principles. Links between homelessness and poor health, including mental health problems, have long been recognised (Scott, 1993). Health, social services and community groups in Liverpool mirrored this national and international recognition of the need to target this group. Local research (Ferran *et al.*, 1993) confirmed that these issues needed addressing in Liverpool. A variety of local services were developed, drawing upon published data and local knowledge. These developments were somewhat piecemeal, but driven forward by product champions, they generated new information, skills and experience. This knowledge base was shared and amplified through reports and a stakeholder conference in 1994 (McCarthy and Odunaiya, 1994). Further revisions and changes continue to be made to the services in the light of developing knowledge.

The criteria listed above were not just met once in this process; they were continually carried forward. The services would not have developed without product champions, but most of the stakeholders involved now, were not involved in the early years, and if the process purely depended on product champions, it would have withered away. Similarly, the nature of the services has had to change to reflect changes in knowledge, need and resources. No-one is likely to suggest that the current services are perfect, but there is wide agreement that they are much more effective, efficient and efficacious than 10 years ago. This is an important reminder that targeting requires a lot of input, and usually quite some time to produce identifiable results. Only by identifying outcomes, and re-evaluating the benefits and costs, can progress be maintained.

To promote targeting that is effective, efficient and efficacious, it is essential that the right approaches be applied to the people most likely to benefit. The present reality is that this sort of targeting is still at an early stage. The increasing coverage of mental health topics by the Cochrane Database, NICE and other organisations will improve the ability of purchasers, therapists and patients to make good treatment choices. It is important that such organisations take into account all types of research. There is a risk that overemphasis could be given to quantitative studies, especially randomised controlled trials. These are definitely the best way of comparing two treatments for evidence of beneficial effect at the population level, but other sorts of research, e.g., qualitative or naturalistic studies, may be more helpful for issues of efficacy and efficiency. Training to make best use of information is essential. It will take a long time for the reviews and guidelines to cover even the common questions. Guidelines and reviews will, by their nature, always lag behind the cutting edge of developments. Search skills and critical appraisal skills, that is, the ability to search for best evidence and to evaluate it, will therefore be necessary to support planning and good clinical services.

Targeting, as set out above, promotes active questioning and goal-setting. This promotes the re-definition of targets linked to ongoing learning, as knowledge increases. This approach also enhances zeal and reduces risk of burnout. Elitism, in the positive sense of promoting the best, is a healthy spin-off. Product champions are necessary to bring attention to the benefits. Too little is made of much good work because it is not recorded and published. Targeting can help to define and refine guidance. Evidence of effectiveness can be included in guidelines that are clinically relevant.

In summary, targeting is an excellent way of maximising the benefit from a given level of resource, *if* the above issues are acknowledged and addressed.

## References

Davidson, I.A. and Cowley, A. (1998), 'The HoST Initiative - Making Targeting Explicit', *RADICAL Annual Report,* North Mersey Community (NHS) Trust, Liverpool.

Department of Health. (1990), *The Care Programme Approach for People with a Mental Illness Referred to the Specialist Psychiatric Services,* HC(90)23, LASSL(90)11, Department of Health, London.

Department of Health (1993), *The Health of the Nation. Key Area Handbook. Mental Illness,* Department of Health, London.

Department of Health (1995), *Building Bridges. A Guide to Arrangements for Inter-Agency Working for the Care and Protection of Severely Mentally Ill People,* Department of Health, London.

Department of Health (1996), *Local Services for People with Mental Health Problems,* Department of Health, London.

Department of Health (1998), *Modernising Mental Health Services: Safe, Sound and Supportive,* The Stationery Office, London.

Department of Health (1999a), *Effective Care Co-ordination in Mental Health Services: A Policy Booklet SSI/NHS Executive,* Department of Health, London.

Department of Health (1999b), *National Service Frameworks: Mental Health,* The Stationery Office, London.

Department of Health (1999c), *Reform of the Mental Health Act 1983: Proposals For Consultation,* (Cm 4480) Department of Health, London.

Ferran, J., O'Shea, B. and Davidson, I.A. (1993), ' The Homeless and the Mental Health Services - a Liverpool Study', *Psychiatric Bulletin,* vol. 17, pp. 649-51.

House of Comons (1983), *The Mental Health Act,* HMSO, London.

McCarthy, J. and Odunaiya, H. (1994), 'Homelessness in Liverpool - Who Cares?' *Radical Innovations,* Vol 1. North Mersey Community (NHS) Trust, Liverpool.

Sackett, D.L., Richardson, W.S., Rosenberg, W., and Haynes, R.B. (1997), *Evidence Based Medicine. How to Practice and Teach EBM,* Churchill-Livingstone, London.

Scally, G. and Donaldson, L.D. (1998), 'Clinical Governance and the Drive for Quality Improvement in the New NHS in England', *British Medical Journal,* vol. 317, pp. 61-5.Scott, J. (1993), ' Homelessness and Mental Illness', *British Journal of Psychiatry,* 162, pp. 314-24.

Scott, J. (1993), ' Homelessness and Mental Illness', *British Journal of Psychiatry,* 162, pp. 314-24.

*Further Reading*

The best U.K. site for exploring evidence based approaches to mental health issues is (www.psychiatry.ox.ac.uk/cebmh).

PubMed (www.ncbi.nih.gov/PubMed/overview.html) is a free internet search facility for Medline. A trained librarian will enhance the quality of the search.

The Department of Health website (www.doh.gov.uk) is an excellent site for up to date DoH circulars and reports.

# 5 A Social Services' Perspective

HELEN SUMNER

## Introduction

Since their inception, social services departments (SSDs) have grappled with the rationing of services. Rationing, although an emotive term, at least contains within it a notion of apportionment, and a rational application of a system of priorities for allocating resources. Targeting, on the other hand, contains within it the notion of a direct application, or 'hit', together with the potential for a random 'fall out', or completely to miss! This opinion-based chapter explores the notion and implication of targeting in mental health from a social services perspective, although no claims are made for it being comprehensive or representative of the views of others working within social care, social work or social services. The author is an Assistant Director of Special Needs and Disability in a local authority SSD. The chapter begins with a brief description of the context and the challenge for SSDs in targeting resources on people with severe and enduring mental illness. Then, the delivery of an appropriate response by SSDs is considered. The chapter is concluded with a discussion suggesting a possible way forward.

## The Context and Challenge

It is frequently and fervently argued that rationing is needed in health and social care, since need is infinite and resources are not. It might also be argued, however, that need is finite. If we assume a notion of perfect mental and physical health, and complete social equilibrium as a finite state beyond which resources need not be spent, then the total amount of necessary resources could theoretically be quantified as necessary to achieve this aim. The real position, though, is that a line has to be drawn in a place that falls short of this nirvana. It is a political and social decision as to who draws the line and where it is placed. tension is played out. Mental health is, arguably, the most complex arena in which this particular tension is played out. It is an area in which it is most difficult to draw the line between what is mental illness, poor mental health, adequate mental health, or a state which falls short of what Maslow (1954) might term full 'self-actualisation'.

Richard Titmus (1963) pointed out that, as a modern society, we note the importance of the definition of 'need'. With the infinite and cumulative processes of social and technological change since the 19th century, the situation of the recognition of need has changed radically, and is affected greatly by rising expectation. If the concept of need is, therefore, ever-evolving and changing, then so must the point at which the above stated line is drawn, since there can be no objective and finite conclusion about its position. Perhaps no-one better sums up the position than Titmus quoting from Durkheim: 'Man becomes, in the pursuit of individual life goals, more aware of his dependency, more viable to failure, more exposed to pain'. This is the overall context in which social care for people with mental health problems and mental illnesses must be sited. Possibly no condition is more subjectively experienced than mental health or illness.

Exhortations to 'target services on those most in need' are, therefore, generally unhelpful in the extreme, unless those involved in providing services have worked to achieve a useful and common understanding of the terms which they are being encouraged to employ. This is further complicated when the priorities of different agencies involved in providing care also differ. That said, clarity in national priority terms is to be welcomed, since it gives agencies a common and clearer focus. Further, it is to be hoped that it provides an opportunity to develop joint strategies that move towards a common goal or target. Achieving the 'bulls eye' can be more difficult, especially where other imperatives are at work. This goal can be difficult when agencies responsible for the provision of social care are hampered in their task by a variety of boundary difficulties, including those of geography, eligibility or culture. If the definition of good mental health is difficult, then this is further compounded when the agencies involved in the provision of care each have their own definition. Targeting can easily become skewed, given that 'depression will affect nearly half of all women and a quarter of all men in the UK before the age of seventy' (DoH, 1998). Changes in public awareness can also lead to what was once seen as part and parcel of the human condition being defined as abnormal in the absence of appropriate social supports.

In summary, there is a definite tension in some areas between the need to target services on those with severe mental illness, who may arguably be those most in need, and the vast majority of people affected by mental health problems. The constituency of the latter runs far and wide, and they are most likely, initially, to turn to their GPs.

**The Social Services Care Response**

How then, can social work and social care respond to the challenge to promote general health and well being, and concentrate their responses on both acute illness and supporting, in the community, people who have intense and specialised needs? I will outline this further below, but first, it is necessary to look in greater depth at the context in which the activity of targeting for good mental health is meant to take place. To do this, we have to turn our attention to the 1980's, although mental health services have been in transition for a good deal longer than this. The shift away from care in asylums has been well documented. Interestingly, the reduction in the number of people in large asylums, due to developments in psychotropic medication and rising aspirations, also led to the relocation of acute admission services to general hospitals, as well as the creation of community services. By the 1990's, market forces had joined the picture. The newly created NHS Trusts were encouraged to seek 'business' from GPs, and were realigning their services in order to be able to respond.

Paradoxically, this occurred at around the same time that government mental health policy demanded the targeting and concentration of activity on people with severe and enduring mental illness. For example, the Mental Health Specific Grant to local authorities was to be spent with the agreement of the relevant health authorities, and focused on the social care of people whose mental illness was so severe that they were in contact with the specialist psychiatric services. Thus, a tension existed. On the one hand, SSDs were required to work in partnership and co-operation with 'health' (which, by now, had become a purchasing and providing entity) in the provision of social care to those with the most severe and enduring mental illness. On the other hand, health Trusts were busy setting about selling their community psychiatric nursing services to GPs. Although the larger volume of Trusts' patients' needs were different to those in the 'target' group, the pressures to respond with solutions were, and continue to be, great. However, the average GP consultation time is unlikely to allow for in-depth counselling.

In numerical terms, the mental health needs of people presenting to GPs tend to be focused on the more general mental illnesses. GPs will see individuals with severe and enduring mental health problems comparatively rarely. GPs will be approached by relatively large numbers of people with reactive illnesses, many of which are self-limiting, and by people who have relationship and social problems, exacerbated by environment and lifestyle factors. The tendency was, therefore, for GPs to purchase community psychiatric nursing care for those people who would not be described as severe and enduringly mentally ill, whilst the SSDs struggled to engage their colleagues in setting up Community Mental Health Teams (CMHTs) to target precisely on this latter client group. The problem persists, and is in no way ameliorated by the creation of the Primary Care Groups (PCGs). The consequence, of course, is that when 'targeted' referrals need to be made, then space may not be available in the busy schedule of the Trust's services. There is some acknowledgement of this dichotomy, illustrated by the work of Patmore and Weaver (1991) on CMHTs. Yet, similar pressures tend to remain. The primary health care modernisation agenda and the emergence of PCGs take the trend further. If GPs, via PCGs and Primary Care Trusts, take a larger role in commissioning mental health services, then these issues will be exacerbated unless the dichotomy can be addressed.

The consequences of the trend described above have been to skew the caseloads of both psychiatric and social care professionals. In 1997, Professor Peter Huxley began research into matching resources to client need. In a number of authorities, analysis of the caseloads of community psychiatric nurses and social workers revealed that the social workers were working with a greater proportion of clients/patients who had the most severe and enduring problems. This finding in no way detracts from the subjective needs of those who have less severe mental health problems. Nevertheless, it does illustrate how a series of conflicting policy objectives has, in some circumstances, led to unintended consequences.

So how has social care met this challenge? Following a series of inquiries, the government laid out its expectations that health and social services would work together to provide a 'seamless service' and target services on those with the most severe and enduring mental illness. At around the same time, the *NHS and Community Care Act* (House of Commons, 1990) established the division of roles between purchaser and provider in health and social care. Care management was introduced, and prescriptive models were drawn up which, it is commonly felt, concentrated on the numerically highest area of demand, mainly that for older people. The care management model, therefore, did not fit in well to the provision of mental health services. In addition, social workers were busy trying to become fully integrated members of CMHTs. Debates raged about the relative, and sometimes contradictory, role of the Approved Social Worker, or the care manager, as purchaser of mental health services, and the social work role as provider of counselling and ongoing support. Various departments have taken different approaches, but the potential contradictions have never been fully resolved. Pressures upon community psychiatric nurse colleagues and others, in terms of the demand for counselling and other services, have further affected the social work role. One of the basic contradictions inherent in the care management model was that it tended to assume shorter-term interventions than normally required for people with long-term and severe mental illness. It assumed a 'throughput' of cases, whereas long-term care for the client group under discussion requires intensive and ongoing support.

Social care can also be affected by targeting in health care. Throughout the 1990's, and in response to the *NHS and Community Care Act* (House of Commons, 1990), the NHS has continued to try to define its responsibilities in respect of continuing care. The Court of Appeal has recently offered some clarity in relation to the case between Pamela Coughlan and North East Devon Health Authority, although it remains to be seen how this will be played out in the mental health arena. Since there was disinclination by the government to issue national guidelines, the discussions in relation to continuing care have had to take place on a local basis between health and social services. There has, therefore, been widespread variation! This has affected social care agencies in their targeting, since the resource implications of the drawing of the line relating to continuing care will impact very largely on social services' responsibilities and resources. If, in turn, social services target their spending on those who are the most severely ill, this 'grey area' is one that will consume most resources, leaving less for the larger group of people who may need or require help.

This particular conundrum also presents a challenge for Joint Commissioning, since the pooling of resources cannot always solve the shortage of resources. Shared priorities in an environment of scarce resources and pressure on provision will tend to encourage agencies to concentrate on provision at the heavy end of the tariff. Relationships between health authorities and SSDs vary across the country, but even where relationships are good and agreements work well in practice, the shift in emphasis by one authority necessarily shifts the emphasis of another. Whilst this is done in a relatively well planned way, the impact of market forces, or of more random purchasing outside a targeting framework, can reap havoc on a rational approach to rationing.

## Concluding Discussion

*Risk Management and Public Safety*

One with a suspicious mind might argue that political exhortations to concentrate services on those people with the most severe and enduring mental illness are influenced by the wider political agenda of public safety and risk elimination. It has been argued, for example, that a lot of what is positive in the government's new mental health agenda is undermined by an over-emphasis on compliance and control. Alongside this, the strand of positive public health promotion cannot co-exist until, and unless, staff working in the mental health services are supported by a wider agenda that acknowledges that tragedies can happen in spite of the most effective, co-ordinated and streamlined services, the focus on prevention will be undermined. However, staff will be forced to concentrate on, and target, the people with the most severe and enduring mental illness, whilst the public safety agenda remains. Issues regarding people who are 'dangerous', who also have a personality disorder, are interesting here. There is a wide amount of disagreement about what constitutes a personality disorder and whether these disorders are treatable. Also, the criminal justice system has traditionally punished people for what they have done, rather than what they might do. This state of affairs may change with the reforms to mental health legislation. It remains to be seen what the role of mental health social services will be in this unfolding agenda.

*The Way Forward?*

So what then might be a solution? It will continue to be difficult for health and social care agencies to attempt to meet both the policy objective of targeting services for those with the greatest need, as well as, on the greater numbers of people who have less severe mental health difficulties. Further, it is arguable that people with 'less severe mental health needs' are accurately described as 'less severe'. One approach to resolving the dilemma facing agencies might be a change in conceptual framework, which draws a much clearer line between what should be the responsibility of the statutory agencies to address, and that which might require more community-orientated responses. It is frequently the case that health, GPs and social workers are drawn into providing care where relationships have broken down and where social problems are a primary cause of mental health problems. Social problems requiring family community support that is missing can escalate into the need for primary care intervention, and if untreated or ameliorated, into the need for secondary care. The prevention agenda is, therefore, an attractive one. Brown *et al.,* (1978) describe this clearly.

Perhaps different responses should be created for different problems. It appears unreasonable to allocate trained and professional community psychiatric nursing or social work resources in situations where tender loving care, or a shoulder to cry on, is required. It does appear that, as a society, we should be looking to recreate, stimulate or support 'community', or provide alternatives to this type of professional care. These 'supporters' could be made aware of mental health issues, trained in symptom recognition, and taught when to refer to others. Generally, they could provide the old type of listening and care which many communities and families have now lost. Where this type of promotion is untenable (and I think this will be rare), additional, more structured support may be constructed in a way that offers real answers to people in need, gives GPs somewhere to refer patients, and grasps the social care agenda. Perhaps a panel of specialised response agencies looking at bereavement, relationship problems and so on could provide an alternative to referral into specialised services in a way that also protects the service for other groups. Only in this way can effective targeting continue to take place on individuals seen as most in need. Primary care might give its attention to this approach.

# References

Brown, G.W. and Harris, T. (1978), *The Social Origins of Depression: A Study of Psychiatric Disorder in Women,* Tavistock, London.

Department of Health (1998), *Modernising Mental Health Services: Safe, Sound and Supportive,* The Stationery Office, London.

House of Commons (1990), *The NHS and Community Care Act,* HMSO, London.

Huxley, P. (1997), *Matching Resources in Mental Health,* Department of Health, London.

Maslow, (1954), *Motivation and Personality,* Harper & Row, London.

Patmore, C. and Weaver, T. (1991), *Community Mental Health Teams: Lessons for Planners and Managers,* Good Practices in Mental Health, London.

Titmuss, R. (1963), *Essays on the Welfare State,* George Allen & Unwin, London.

# 6 A General Practitioner's Perspective

ROBERT WYN EDWARDS

## Introduction

Severe Mental Illness (SMI) registers have recently been established in virtually all general practices in Wirral as part of a strategy to raise the profile of this patient group. This chapter is written from the perspective of a Wirral GP. It reflects his thoughts regarding use of the SMI register, with particular regard to how it has affected the practice. It is a three partner non-fundholding urban practice in the centre of Birkenhead, with a list size of 5,000 patients. It has higher than average numbers of children and young adults, and lower than average numbers of the elderly on the list. The practice covers a moderately deprived area with higher than average levels of psychiatric morbidity. The population served also has high levels of alcoholism and drug abuse. The opinions expressed in this chapter represent a fairly personal view shared by some, but not all, other general practitioners. It has been shaped by many different factors.

## The Primary Care Context

Psychiatry has always been something of a Cinderella speciality, and has always found difficulty in attracting adequate funding. This may be because it seems to be given a low priority, both by doctors and by the public (including politicians!). It often falls to enthusiastic individuals or pressure groups to lobby for greater resources. In fact, the amount of resources spent on mental health varies greatly from area to area.

General Practitioners also vary tremendously in their enthusiasm and ability in the subject. Most will not have undergone any postgraduate training, since it is not an essential part of GP training. A GP's experience will also be influenced by where he or she practices; an inner city practitioner will inevitably have to deal with a larger psychiatric caseload than a colleague in a suburban or rural practice. Often one finds that, in a practice of several doctors, one practitioner will be seen by the patients as being more sympathetic and will draw a disproportionate percentage of the psychiatric workload. However, one advantage of this is that this GP would become more familiar with psychiatric drugs; more proficient in prescribing; and, generally, more experienced and proficient in treating psychiatric cases. GPs are often criticised for prescribing sub-therapeutic doses of tricyclic antidepressants, and this would be more likely from a less experienced doctor.

A GP has various options when presented with mental health problems. These are influenced by various factors, such as the GP's experience and knowledge and, also, by access to other resources such as psychiatrists, community psychiatric nurses (CPNs), psychologists, counsellors and social workers. It is this mix of resources which has altered over the years, and has altered again following the implementation of the SMI registers locally.

**Historical Factors**

A number of changes over the past few years have altered the way we manage our mental health patients in primary care. One major change up to now has been our referral patterns. If we felt we could not manage a patient ourselves, we would refer on to a psychiatrist. The psychiatrist would then see the patient, commence treatment, and probably refer to other mental health workers such as CPNs. Up to about ten years ago, CPNs were not accessible from primary care. The 1970s and 1980s also saw a large shift of psychiatric patients out of the old style asylums and into the community. The number of psychiatric beds dropped dramatically, to the extent that in some areas there are now insufficient in-patient facilities. Following on from these developments, in the 1990s there were more changes. CPNs made a conscious bid to be more autonomous. They became accessible from primary care, and as a result possibly of taking direct referrals from GPs, became far more involved in treating patients with less severe illness such as depression, anxiety states and phobias. At this time there were many innovative schemes often involving CPNs offering clinic sessions in GP surgeries.

The other big change was the advent and growth of fundholding. This represented a huge change in how health services were delivered, and was part of the concept of splitting the health service into providers and purchasers. At the time it was a very controversial policy of which most doctors, including the BMA, disapproved. However, by 1997 half of all

GPs were involved in some form of fundholding. Opinion amongst GPs regarding the value of fundholding still varies considerably, but personally I believe that it lead to a two-tier primary care service. With respect to mental health, fundholders were able to use their budgets to fund various schemes. Many employed counsellors and also purchased mental health services from the local providers to have in-house sessions from CPNs and psychologists, when non-fundholders did not enjoy such extra facilities. There then often existed a situation where patients of fundholders had short waits to see one of these staff, while non-fundholders had to endure long waiting times for their patients, although services were often provided by the same Trust. However, the present Labour Government eventually dismantled fundholding with effect from the 1st of April 1999. It was replaced by Primary Care Groups (PCGs), which will be discussed later.

By the mid-1990s, fundholding was flourishing, with more practices signing up each year, mainly because they wished not to be left behind. CPNs were enjoying more autonomy and were seeing a wider range of mental health problems. Also, there had been a rapid expansion of the use of counsellors to treat people with anxiety, neurotic depression and other minor, but acute, problems. Counselling has became phenomenally successful. In the mid-1980s, very few practices used counsellors but, recently, they have become an essential part of the primary care team. There are several reasons for this. Firstly, there was a groundswell of opinion starting in the late 1980s that anyone suffering a mentally traumatic event should be offered counselling. This relatively new idea rapidly became accepted as the norm, and patients often now approach their doctor requesting such help. Another possible factor is that GPs have become increasingly busy with paperwork and duties other than seeing patients. They have, therefore, been happy to delegate some of their anxious and depressed patients to counsellors. Patients were generally happy to see a counsellor as the counsellor could devote a lot more time to them.

Around this time, there were several high profile homicides committed by schizophrenic patients, where it was felt that their care had fallen short of what should be expected. There was also disquiet at the pace of change in the secondary sector, where patients were being actively moved back into the community, seemingly without adequate resources. It was felt, for various reasons, that some patients with major illness were not being adequately treated. Some were slipping through the net and were not being picked up by anyone; others were known about by the GP, but no one else. CPNs were spending more time with less severely ill patients, which inevitably gave less time to the more severely ill. As a result a general rethink was suggested with the aim of targeting resources more effectively to those who really needed them. This sounds good in theory, but does it work in practice?

## Local History

Policy changed locally in 1997 when SMI registers were first set up. These registers were kept within each general practice in the district, and listed all patients within the practice who had a severe or enduring mental illness. A pathway of referrals was suggested to get patients to appropriate services. Following the implementation of the registers, these became the core workload of the CPNs. In fact, a target was set that 80% of their caseloads were to be on the register. Patients with lesser problems, who were deemed not suitable for CPNs, were to be referred to a practice-based counsellor (which the Trust also provided to all practices). If the patient had more complex problems, then a referral to psychology was suggested.

On a superficial level this model looked fine and even logical. I think, given time and adequate resources, it would work well. However, in practice, it caused a lot of difficulties, some still not resolved. I think that there were several reasons for this. Firstly, was there any need for change? I have outlined above the reasons why the Government wished to change the way CPNs worked. However, there was a lot of feeling locally that what had gradually evolved over time was working perfectly well without any obvious deficiencies. In other words "If it ain't broke, why fix it?" The change was also implemented in some practices in a very radical way, which, coupled with problems in other areas, caused quite a lot of problems for some GPs.

Secondly, perhaps the biggest problem was agreeing throughout the area who should be on the SMI register in the first place. When the registers were first set up it became obvious that there were huge variations between them, which threatened to make a mockery of the whole exercise. The registers were set up by the CPN attached to the practice along with the GPs. Due to a variety of factors each practice came up with their own view as to who should be on them! On one extreme, some practices only included patients with a psychotic illness, whilst others included everyone who had had a major tranquilliser. There then followed several meetings to try and resolve this problem and come up with a more prescriptive definition to achieve some kind of standardisation. The decision reached was that patients with a psychotic illness, and those with major neuroses which significantly hampered their day-to-day lives and had endured for more than six months, should go on the register. This would include patients with learning disability and those with co-existing drug abuse (dual diagnosis) who also satisfy the criteria for entry. I think this is probably the best definition we can get, but even this has an element of ambiguity in that the exact diagnosis and the severity of any disability are hard to quantify in any objective way. Inclusion on the register is, therefore, often reliant on the perception of the individual GP seeing the patient, and we all have slightly different ideas as to what 'SMI' means. Hence, registers in different practices will probably have slightly differing criteria for inclusion. Furthermore, as these registers are held in practices and are 'owned' by them, the only way to ensure standardisation is to have a person (who could it be?) to go around all the practices and check them. Up to now that would have proved a difficult problem. However, with the development of PCGs, this could be achieved through clinical governance in that a doctor is now appointed or elected by colleagues to look at clinical standards within a PCG. I feel that practices would be happy for such a doctor to look critically at their SMI registers and comment if any changes need to be made.

Thirdly, problems immediately arose following the change because patients with distressing symptoms of anxiety, depression or phobias, who had previously seen a CPN, found themselves on long waiting lists to see a counsellor or psychologist. These patients felt rather unloved, even abandoned by the health service and left their GPs feeling rather frustrated and annoyed by the whole situation. This leads on to another important factor. As GPs, we see an ever increasing number of patients with distressing symptoms of anxiety or depression, often related to increasing family break-ups, unemployment and poverty. Many of these patients prove very hard to manage and take up a lot of time; they are usually far more problematic to us than those whose schizophrenia has stabilised. It is these patients, with common mental disorders, whom we need help in managing - help which is now harder to access.

Another worry I have is that when we see a new patient with mental health problems, we have to make a careful assessment as to what the diagnosis is and who to refer to. Sometimes we may get it wrong, and whereas in the past someone else would see the patient (usually a CPN) and perhaps pick up on this fairly quickly, this is often no longer the case. The government has the goal of reducing the suicide rate as one of its *Health of the Nation* (DoH, 1992) and *Saving Lives* (DoH, 1999) targets, and I wonder if this change is really going to help that?

## Ongoing Changes

In 1997 a Labour Government was elected which has duly carried out its pledge to scrap fundholding. It officially came to an end on the 31st of March 1999. In its place was the PCG, short for Primary Care Group, which encompassed all GPs in a specific area. The GPs elect about six of their colleagues to sit on a board, which also includes representatives from various other bodies such as nurses, pharmacists, social services and lay members. This has brought in a feeling of increased equity between practices, and much of the work undertaken this year has been the de-commissioning of fundholding, coupled with spreading any extra services offered by fundholding practices to cover all the practices involved. This will take time, but I am sure that it will eventually be achieved. Over the next couple of years or so most PCGs, whether they like it or not, probably will develop into Primary Care Trusts (PCTs). In effect, these will be like mini health authorities which will directly purchase services on behalf of their patients including, of course, mental health services. It will be interesting to see whether mental health funding will improve or not, in terms of percentage of total health expenditure. What will eventually happen is that GPs will have more influence over how money is spent in various areas of healthcare, and the hope is that if there are any areas which are underfunded, or need extra funding, then action could be taken to correct matters. Of course mental health services will be among many vying for the PCG board's attention. Mental health has not done well in the past; it remains to be seen if it will fare better under PCGs or PCTs.

## Conclusion

I have put forward my various thoughts about mental health services and how the introduction of SMI registers has affected them. Like many ideas which may appear to be worthwhile on paper but often don't work out so well in practice, up to now this appears to be another example.

I would agree that in practice it is a very sensible way of reorganising mental health services, targeting appropriate care to the patient. It has not worked too well, I feel, because the service was stretched already at the time the registers were introduced, with numbers of CPNs below optimum levels. It also exposed the fact that psychiatry is underfunded, both locally and nationally. This general lack of funding was also exacerbated by inequity between practices regarding the provision of counsellors and in-house CPN clinics, depending on whether a practice was fundholding or not.

However, I do now feel optimistic that matters will improve, and as a consequence the use of SMI registers will become useful and practical. In summary, for the system to work properly, a patient following a consultation with the GP should be seen by one of the psychiatric team within a reasonable time. This would be the same day for an urgent problem, within a week if referred to a CPN, soon after referral to a counsellor for assessment (followed by a wait of no longer than 6 weeks for the full counselling work) and within 3 months if referred to a psychologist, again following an initial assessment. I feel that if all these factors were in place, the SMI registers could be implemented successfully, and would be a useful tool for appropriate care to be concentrated on the most needy patients.

## References

Department of Health (DoH) (1992) *The Health of the Nation*. Cm. 1986, HMSO, London.
Department of Health (DoH) (1999) *Saving Lives: Our Healthier Nation*. Cm. 4386, The Stationery Office, London.

# 7 A Service User's Perspective

PAUL GOLDING

## Introduction

Some time ago, I was asked to join the Advisory Group for the SEMI Registers Project that was being set up in the Wirral. The Advisory Group was made up of various stakeholders involved in establishing primary care-held registers across the Wirral, together with the team who were conducting the research to monitor and evaluate this process. The research project was looking at whether or not the keeping of registers in primary care of those suffering from severe and enduring mental illness (SEMI) would lead to an improvement in their care and quality of life. The intention was that this would be achieved by targeting people with SEMI, along with the type, appropriateness and co-ordination of the services (health, social and voluntary) provided to them.

So why was I asked to join this group, and what special skills did I bring to it? Well, I have seen life from both sides of the fence. I have suffered from a major mental illness for most of my adult life, spent time in hospital as an in-patient, lived in a semi-residential home for 14 months, and attended a day centre for people with mental illness for four years. I was instrumental in setting up and chairing a mental health charity on the Wirral. After this, I went to work for Sefton social services department as a Mental Health Development Officer for one year. I am currently working for Wallasey Citizen's Advice Bureau as a Specialist Advisor on Welfare Benefits, and as an Outreach Worker for the local Mental Health Resource Unit. Throughout this time, I have remained closely involved with service user, and ex-service user, groups on the Wirral, especially the Wirral Mental Health Forum. The committee of the Mental Health Forum thought that another person and myself should be their representatives on the SEMI Registers Advisory Group and provide a service user perspective. Through my involvement in the SEMI Registers Advisory Group, and because of the link between the SEMI Research Project and this book, I was asked to write a chapter. In this chapter, I was asked to put down some of my experiences, thoughts and opinions about targeting people with SEMI, including my thoughts about what is appropriate in terms of a quality service.

It seems to me that the caring profession is often tied to looking at

131

diagnosis, rather than how disabled a person is. Perhaps we need to look at what can be done to treat the individual and tailor their treatment to them, taking account of what has brought this person to where they are right now. There are good ways of finding out people's needs and whether those needs are being met, or not. However, meeting those needs has to be multi-disciplinary in approach, and must look at achievable goals in the short, medium and long-term. This process must not be directive on the part of the professionals, but should involve the individual.

In this chapter, I will discuss some of the long-standing issues in mental health that are in danger of being made worse, especially for people with SEMI. I will begin with some background on how, historically, people with mental illness have been treated by society. I will talk about the effects of stigma and discrimination on the lives of people with SMI. Then, I will consider the relationship between power and treatment of serious mental illness. Next, I will focus on the public health and primary care agendas for mental health, and how these relate to the individual attending their GP's surgery. Finally, I will conclude with a brief discussion of some of the points I have raised, and my thoughts about the future for mental health services.

## Background

Throughout history people with mental illness have been stigmatized and marginalized by society. In my view, this tendency has increased over the last few years, as the care of people with mental illness has become more of an issue in the public consciousness. Since the Zito affair, there have been a number of knee-jerk reactions to the long-term care of people with SEMI on the part of the government. Suddenly, through the media accounts, the public became aware that there were large numbers of very psychotic people out in the community who were dangerous. There developed a quest to safeguard society from the people with SEMI. However, what this type of reaction does is to make people with SEMI, who are trying to live in the community, feel frightened that the so-called 'caring community' is really the long arm of authority. This authority wants to subdue them, by seeking to increase their medication, or take away more of their rights. Put simply, it seems to many that we live in a society that does not care; a society that only starts to look for answers when things go wrong.

What has been provided by means of goods and services for people with SEMI in real terms since the inception of the *Community Care Act*? A good quality of service for people with mental illness has been found to be lacking because of the unwillingness of local and national government to invest in proper care. People with mental illness are not allowed the same opportunities to goods and services as the rest of the community, such as having a mortgage or a bank account. If they do have one of these, they may have it taken out of their control because of their mental health problems. Another common experience for people with mental illness is getting into debt because of pressure to enter into credit agreements, or to make arrangements to extend their credit, or to agree to make payments that they are never going to be able to meet. This aspect of the world of finance and consumerism is an area that can cause a person with a mental health problems to worry to the extent that their condition worsens.

All too often we hear of how people with mental illness are left with no basic amenities and no ability to pay for heating and food, for one reason or another. Every winter, as a person who has worked as an advocate for the last 7 years, I have listened to how some people with SEMI keep warm by sitting wrapped up in a quilt in the dark with no food. This may be because the benefits agency has refused to give them a crisis loan, they have lost their money (again), the gas or electricity company have disconnected their supply, or social services have not been able to give them any food vouchers, and so on. Many service users who are eligible for certain benefits find that the way the benefits agency works means that they are unable to apply without specialist help (e.g. Disability Living Allowance). Now, with the announcement of the government's reforms, we are told that the mental health service is to be modernised – to become 'safe, sound and supportive' - but for whom?

**Stigma and Discrimination**

It is interesting to note that when you talk to differing sections of society about who they see as most in need of resources, the physically disabled are the ones thought to be most in need, especially if they are children. Further, some people in the disabled community believe in a hierarchy of disablement, in which people with mental illness are at the bottom. With this in mind, how can we expect to change society's attitude to people with mental illness, given the ingrained perception that they are not worthy, or less worthy, of our care and compassion? When you have a physical illness you are diagnosed as having this or that wrong with you. On the other hand, if you have a mental illness and are put in front of three or four psychiatrists, the chances are they will come up with different diagnoses. This assessment will be visited on you because of your actions, and your freedom will depend on how soon you can show that you are able to live a normal life, and that your behaviour is not determined by the identified condition.

In recent years there has been a rise in various forms of discrimination against people with SEMI, not by professional people working with this group in the community (and that has been about for many years), but by society, the media and the government. Oppressive behaviour is used either directly, or indirectly, towards an individual or group of people, with the result that they are marginalised, ridiculed, belittled, or otherwise harmed. Despite this, the government's mental health policy clearly states that public safety is the first priority, although it also claims to want to stamp out discrimination. What does this prioritisation say about people with SEMI? I am fully aware that the government will say there is current legislation covering all types of discrimination and bad practices that people with mental illness may come across. However, as yet, there has been no successful application made under the *Disability Discrimination Act* by anyone with a mental illness. Also, fear of discrimination prevents people with SEMI from being able to walk over their front door step without worrying that they are going to be singled out in some way, or beaten up because they are considered dangerous. Or, if they return home, they may realistically worry whether their property has been broken into and their belongings stolen. If such an incident is reported to the police, it has been some people's experience that a less-than-co-operative constable arrives, who has been there before and knows that the person reporting the crime has a history of mental illness, and appears to just 'go through the motions'.

Discrimination against people with SEMI is also linked to the situations experienced by them – they are discriminated against in terms of being excluded in various ways, expected to live in substandard housing, and not being in receipt of the correct benefits. If they are in employment, they are expected to work long hours for very low wages, because they are told that they should count themselves lucky to be in a job. It should also be noted that many social services departments throughout the country exploit people with mental illness in this way by encouraging people with mental illness to work in sheltered work schemes. They then satisfy their souls by arguing that, if they were paid more, it would have an effect on people's benefits. Will 'Welfare to Work' and the 'New Deal' change all this in the way the government suggests?

## Power and Treatment

Among the powers that statutory agencies have is the power to lock someone up if they are in danger of spreading a contagious disease. I often wonder what would happen if the Minister of Health told these agencies to lock up all those people who have AIDS, or those who are HIV positive, because of the potential and significant risk that anyone who has these conditions poses to the rest of society. Quite rightly there would be an outcry that the government is denying these people the right to live free and independent lives. So what makes people with mental illness so different? Both will need medical treatment from time to time, but don't we all? I am not advocating that people with mental illness should be allowed to deteriorate. I am arguing that the way people are treated does not need to be so oppressive that we end up in a situation where many people leave it until it is too late before they seek help. How will the government address this issue? How will their reforms to the *Mental Health Act* affect this?

To date, the options discussed in relation to mental health have included compulsory Community Treatment Orders, the tagging of people with mental illness, and the re-opening of the asylums. What do these options have to offer? NOTHING! They offer much the same as other draconian measures of the past - another form of authoritarian control of people with SEMI. Historically, this is 'more of the same'. If a patient does not comply, all such an approach achieves is to create mentally disordered offenders. Why can we not learn from the past?

When looking at recovery from any mental illness, we must consider all the available options, including medication and other treatments. But, we must look at the negative side of these treatments, e.g. the use of electro-convulsive therapy. Does this barbaric practice still have any place in modern medicine? Granted, there are some people with SEMI who are a danger in some way, but involving the right services, providing support, training professionals, and the ensuring people can consult their doctors without fear is the way forward. In terms of treatment, I would advocate using the least invasive option. This may mean abandoning some drugs that cause terrible side effects. It may also means funding and making available the newer, more effective drugs that are on the market. Some will say that, if left to their own devices, people with mental illness will choose to do nothing, as this may seem the safest option from their perspective. Well, as a person who has been there, I can say that I did not take the soft option and stay in the sickness role, as many doctors said I would. I confronted my condition when I could, and I still do. It is important to remember that people with SEMI are not unlike any other group of ill people in being able to overcome very disabling conditions with support and the right kind of treatment. Like all illness, depending on what is wrong with you, how your illness is tackled will dictate the period of recovery.

## Mental Illness, Public Health and Primary Care

The government's policy is to prioritise mental health in order to provide better quality of care. While there are no easily agreed definitions of SEMI, what is agreed is that there does exist an inequality and inequity that contributes significantly to ill health and mental ill health. This inequality and inequity is based on differences in power and material wealth. The public health perspective to reduce such underlying inequalities, especially 'for the worst off in society', is very welcome news for mental health. Primary care is seen as being about more than just medical care, and the role of the environment, social and lifestyle factors are recognised to be important in understanding health and illness. The community is seen as having an integral part to play in ensuring that issues are addressed which affect people's health.

However, from an individual perspective, when my general practitioner shows me the surgery's new information leaflet about what is being provided by them in terms of mental health services, it does not tell me what I want to know. It does not tell me how much is being spent on providing a community mental health nurse, why we need to have a psychologist three or four days a week, or why my doctor does not have access to a more relevant method of supplying a fully integrated support system that I can use when I need it. It does not give me information on benefits, how I can access better housing, where I can find someone I can talk to about my claim for Disability Living Allowance, someone who KNOWS what they are talking about. It does not tell me where I can find someone who can offer me real advice on how to negotiate with creditors that does not involve me having to go to someone who, instead of showing me how to do these things, will take over and do it their way without my involvement. Both social services and the health trusts always hold up such services as advocacy, and other such support, as being user-led. However, it has been my experience that these services start out being run by people who do know what it is like to be a service user, but soon lose touch and end up in providing a service they want or, even worse, that the statutory agencies think the service users want. This is often dictated by the restraints of the local authority budget. Will health and social services be willing to allow people to buy in their own care rather than then expecting them to take what is on offer? For those who wish to do this, it would be a truly user-led form of service provision.


**Concluding Thoughts**

It is worth remembering that the vast majority of people, whether they have a serious mental illness or not, want to be left alone to live their own lives. They do not want someone looking over their shoulder, like a band of harpies waiting for them to make a mistake. So why do we as a society continue to do this to only one section of the community by utilizing any and every method we deem necessary to control them? This is as abusive as locking them away in asylums. In the final analysis, we as a society need to educate the public that people with SEMI are not the dangerous individuals that the media (and now the government) seem to make out, but are people who are ill.

For good mental health, people need to be free from discrimination. They need the same rewards of work and a decent home that we all need. Agencies involved in mental health service provision need to ensure that we, as a society, respond to the changing needs that people with SEMI have in their lives. To do this, they must look at ways to involve people with SEMI in the development of services, and to recognise the individual as a valued member of society who is able to contribute. This way, the things that affect the fears, safety and security of people with SEMI can begin to be addressed. Only then can we begin to reverse some of the trends that are evident in mental health and start to provide services that are both used and effective.

It would be a good target to aim for by the end of the next century if we could stop writing about how we can look after people with mental illness, and just do it. It does not take much imagination to know that what we need to do is care. If the provisions that society has in place for people with mental illness have a positive effect in helping them to live a more rewarding life, one in which their needs are met and where they are integrated into the community, then we would be that much closer to good quality, safe services for all. If this is not the case, we continue to fail people with SEMI and then to blame them.

# PART 3
# RESEARCH STUDIES IN TARGETING

# 8 Identifying the Needs of People with Severe Enduring Mental Illness: A Population Approach

ANN HOSKINS

## Introduction

This chapter explores a population approach to identifying the needs of people in the community with severe enduring mental illness (SEMI). The chapter is based on a study carried out in general practice, which identified people with SEMI and the services they accessed. Several issues were highlighted that need to be considered when planning services for this client group. The author is a public health physician who has worked in several urban health districts and, throughout, has maintained an interest in the provision of services for people with mental health problems, especially in the community setting.

## Severe Enduring Mental Illness in the Primary Care Setting

Over the last 10 years, the Department of Health has highlighted the importance of targeting people with SEMI. This policy has arisen partly as a consequence of several high profile inquiries which identified poor quality, uncoordinated services, and the need to reassure the public about the safety of care in the community for this client group. The *National Service Framework* for mental health sets national standards and service models in seven areas, and effective services for people with severe mental illness are given high priority in this document (DoH, 1999).

Primary Care Groups/Trusts (PCG/Ts) will have an important role in determining the services for people with SEMI, both through providing services directly in general practice, and through commissioning services from specialised mental health service providers. If PCG/Ts are to

undertake their new role effectively, it is important that they understand the extent of the problem in their population.
The PCG/Ts will need to:

- identify the number of people with SEMI;
- understand present service usage (both in general practice and specialist services); and,
- identify gaps/areas for enhanced service provision.

There is a wealth of information held in general practice about the morbidity of the practice population. This information, however, is often hard to access as it is held in the form of paper records. The majority of practices are now computerized, although in most cases the computers are used for administration and prescriptions (Sullivan and Mitchell, 1995). An increasing minority of practices use their computers extensively and record all patient information and consultations. However, even in these practices, the use of the computer during the consultation is overestimated by the GPs (Richards *et al.*, 1998). A recent study in the South West of England found that 91% of practices had a desktop computer in their consulting room. Of these, 98% used the computer to look up patient details or prescribe medication; 75% entered details about selected problems; and, only 35% entered information about the patient's presenting problem at every consultation (Watkins *et al.*, 1999). A national pilot into the collection of health data from general practice has supported practices in projects across England to collect data in a uniform way so that comparisons can be made between practices within the project area and with different parts of the country (CHDGP Project Team, 2000).

There have been studies in general practice specifically looking at people with SEMI. A study in practices in the South West Thames area (from a range of inner city to rural settings), identified 90% of long-term mentally ill patients through practice data, and the other 10% through specialized mental health services (Kendrick *et al.*, 1994). A more comprehensive understanding of the number of people with SEMI will, therefore, be obtained from a combination of information from general practice and the specialized mental health services. It is likely that the information from general practice will give a fuller picture of the extent of the problem, as not all people with SEMI will be in touch with specialist mental health services. There will also be a few people with SEMI who are not in touch with either service, especially in urban areas.

**The Study**

*Background*

This chapter draws on work from the Primary Care Data Project in Wirral health district. This project was funded by Wirral Health Authority, and managed jointly by the Department of Public Health and the Medical Audit Advisory Group (MAAG). The public health physician designed the study in consultation with local GPs and psychiatrists. Mental health had a high priority in the district. The mental health strategy, which specified a community-based service, was in the process of being implemented. Mental health services, which used to be managed by the acute trust, had recently moved to the community trust. The health authority and the GPs were interested to identify the levels of SEMI across the district and access to community-based services.

*The Sample*

At the time of this project, the district was divided into six localities based on areas of similar socio-economic conditions. GPs in the localities were involved in locality commissioning with the health authority. The Primary Care Data Project was a network of six 'sentinel practices' - one from each locality. The practices were chosen because their practice population had a similar age/gender and socio-economic profile to that of their locality, and because they were interested in using their computers for clinical data collection. This is not a random sample of practices and, therefore, it is not valid to make statistical extrapolation to the Wirral population. Six practice data analysts (PDAs) worked in each of the practices collecting morbidity information from the practice computers, or case notes, depending on the issue that was being examined. The PDAs collated data in a uniform way, and thus ensured data quality within the practice, and consistency with the other practices involved in the project. This study into severe enduring mental illness is based on one year's data, from July 1995 to June 1996, and covers the six practices.

For the purposes of this study, SEMI is defined as:

- schizophrenia/ schizo-affective disorder; or
- manic depressive psychosis; or

- recurrent depression, where depression has been treated for more than 12 months (part of which occurred in 1994), and/or more than two episodes of depression requiring treatment in the last 5 years.

This definition does not, however, indicate the level of disability the person suffers from their illness. The study examines the care offered in general practice, and the relationship between general practice and specialized mental health services, for this group of people. People with SEMI who are not registered with primary care are not included in the study.

*Objectives*

The main objective is to examine the provision of care to individuals in the practice with SEMI.

Specific objectives are to:

1.  identify those people (16-64 years) with SEMI in each practice;
2.  examine the number of contacts with primary care in the last 12 months;
3.  examine the reasons for contact with primary care i.e. for physical health or mental health problems;
4.  identify the people in contact with the community mental health team in the last 12 months; and,
5.  for people in contact with the mental health team:

    - to ascertain if there is a named key worker identifiable in the notes; and,
    - to identify who has been admitted to hospital.

**Methods**

The core data set and criteria for identifying people with SEMI were drawn up and PDAs were asked to confirm the study details with their respective GPs.

The search for people with SEMI involved the following processes:

- practice computer systems were used to produce initial lists of people with SEMI based on diagnostic coding, drugs prescribed, injections administered and psychiatric referrals;
- medical records were checked manually to eliminate individuals who did not meet the selection criteria;
- PDAs asked GPs for a list of known cases in the last 12 months; and,
- other sources of information included: contact with community psychiatric nurse; contact with social services; and, referral lists held in secondary care.

PDAs were asked to verify their data by checking a 10% sample of patients in the study. In 5 of the practices the sample only needed minor amendments but, in one practice, it was obvious there had been some difficulty with data collection and the study was repeated under the supervision of the coordinator. The data collected were analyzed centrally and the preliminary findings presented to participating practices for verification and comment.

## Results

*Practice Characteristics*

The practice population ranged from 5,876 to 9,994. There was a mixture of fundholding and non-fundholding practices, fundholding practices tending to be in the more deprived areas of the district (the opposite trend was seen nationally). There were 32,716 adults in the16-64 age group, representing 69% of the participating practice population. The practice population for this age group ranged from 3,819 to 7,172.

*People with SEMI Identified through General Practice and Specialized Mental Health Services*

The total number of people with SEMI was 440. Ninety eight percent of these were identified from general practice records; only 0.5% were identified solely through the specialized mental health services; and, for the remaining 1.5%, there was no record. The percentage identified solely from general practice varied by diagnosis: chronic depression, 60% (260), manic depression, 9% (37), and schizophrenia, 31% (135).

*Prevalence of SEMI by Practice and Diagnosis*

Across the six practices the prevalence of SEMI was 13.4/1,000 practice population (aged 16 – 64). The rate varied from 8.7 in locality E to 20.2 in locality B (Table 8.1). Levels of each diagnosis seemed to be related to:

- levels of morbidity in the community and peoples' choice of practice;
- the presence of hostels or other Care in the Community schemes; and,
- GPs' diagnostic and treatment preferences, especially for the people with chronic depression.

*Consultation Rates in General Practice*

The number of contacts with the GP varied by diagnosis, as shown in Figure 8.1. People with chronic depression tended to see their GP most often. Eight percent of people diagnosed with schizophrenia had not seen their GP in the last year. The overall consultation rate was 8.4 per annum. This varied by diagnosis and by practice (Table 8.2).

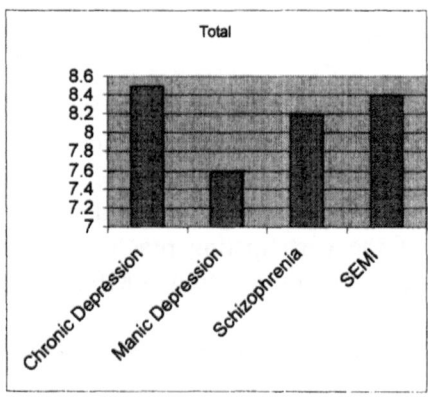

**Figure 8.1  Consultation rates: average number of consultations in preceding 12 months per person by diagnosis**

Table 8.1 Number (rate per 1,000) of people with SEMI by locality and diagnosis

| Locality | A | B | C | D | E | F | Total |
|---|---|---|---|---|---|---|---|
| Chronic Depression | 48(10.3) | 99(13.8) | 27(5.1) | 28(5.6) | 19(2.8) | 45(11.8) | 266(8.1) |
| Schizophrenia | 15(3.2) | 39(5.4) | 25(4.7) | 19(3.8) | 32(4.8) | 7(1.8) | 137(4.2) |
| Manic Depression | 3(0.6) | 7(1.0) | 10(1.9) | 5(1.0) | 7(1.0) | 5(1.3) | 37(1.1) |
| Total SEMI | 66(14.1) | 145(20.2) | 62(11.7) | 52(10.3) | 58(8.7) | 57(14.9) | 440(13.4) |

**Table 8.2  Consultation rates: average number of consultations in preceding 12 months per person by diagnosis and locality**

| Locality | Total | A | B | C | D | E | F |
|---|---|---|---|---|---|---|---|
| Chronic Depression | 8.5 | 8.1 | 7.5 | 13 | 7.6 | 9.5 | 8.7 |
| Manic Depression | 7.6 | 2.7 | 5 | 9.2 | 7.8 | 12.7 | 3.8 |
| Schizophrenia | 8.2 | 6.1 | 7.8 | 9.7 | 5.5 | 10.3 | 8.3 |
| Total SEMI | 8.4 | 6.6 | 7.5 | 11 | 6.8 | 10.3 | 8.2 |

*Reasons for Contact with GP in Preceding 12 months*

The reasons for contact with the GP were obtained from the notes – see Figures 8.2, 8.3 and 8.4. In these figures *major physical illness* included life-threatening illnesses, e.g. myocardial infarction; *minor physical illness* included colds, flu, sprains and sore throats. The mental health problem category was used only when a reference to the mental state was written in the notes. Repeat prescriptions were only included if the GP saw the person. If there was more than one reason for contact written in the notes, both were included in the results.

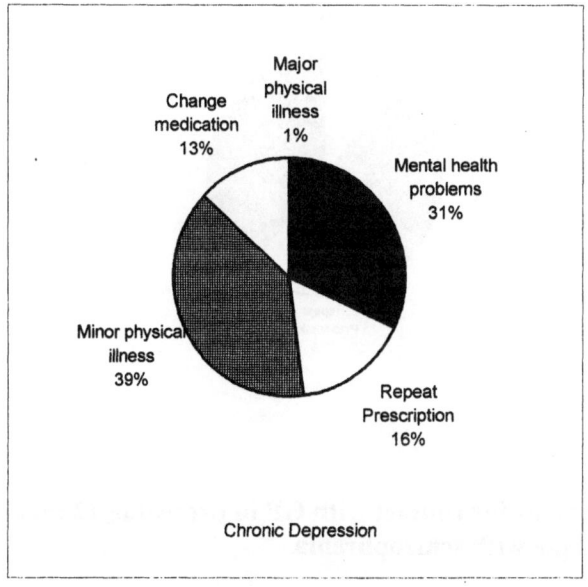

Chronic Depression

**Figure 8.2  Reasons for contact with GP in preceding 12 months in
people with chronic depression**

*Contact with Secondary Care*

Contact with secondary care is illustrated in Table 8.3. Any reference in the GP notes to contact with a secondary care practitioner during the study period was recorded as a contact. This included both letters from the psychiatrist, the CPN, and references to such contact made by the GP in the notes. The Community Trust was also asked to identify with whom they were in contact from the study practices. It should be noted that it was not possible to ascertain from GP notes the type or number of contacts with secondary care professionals. Contact with CPNs was especially difficult to ascertain.

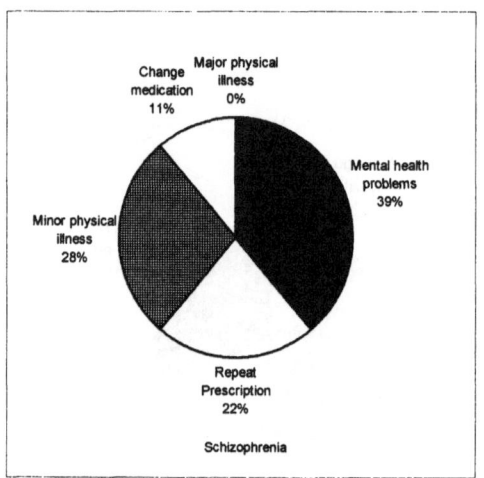

**Figure 8.3  Reasons for contact with GP in preceding 12 months in people with schizophrenia**

The percentage of people who were in contact with specialist mental health services in the preceding 12 months varied by practice (77% to 40%), and diagnosis (schizophrenia, 83%; manic depression, 76%; and chronic depression, 55%). The key worker was only identified in 43% of the notes. This varied by diagnosis (schizophrenia 50%, chronic depression 39%, and manic depression 29%).

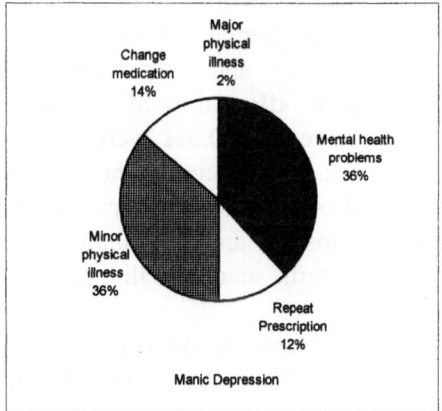

**Figure 8.4  Reasons for contact with GP in preceding 12 months in people with manic depression**

*Admission to Hospital*

Seventy-nine people with SEMI (18%) were admitted to psychiatric hospital during the study year. This varied by diagnosis: schizophrenia 40 (29%), manic depression 9 (24%), and chronic depression 30 (11%). Included in those who experienced admission, 54 (69%) were admitted once, 16 (21%) twice, and one patient was admitted six times in the study period.

**Discussion**

This study has examined the prevalence of SEMI in primary care and has recorded contacts with both primary and secondary care. Definitions of SEMI are problematic, as exemplified in this study by chronic depression. The definition used for chronic depression was chosen as a way of identifying those who are suffering from severe depression. One of the criteria was the use of medication for 12 months – the actual dose prescribed was not assessed. A criticism of using this definition is that in some instances it may represent inadequately treated depression, rather than chronic depression *per se*. The degree of disability experienced by the person was not captured in the study, and could form the basis of further work. In this study, 98% of people affected by SEMI were identified from information held in primary care, and 0.5% were identified solely via specialist mental health services. This is consistent with the study quoted earlier in practices in South West Thames (Kendrick *et al.*, 1994), and a similar project in Liverpool (Hoskins and Langshaw, 1995), where 90% and 93% respectively of long-term mentally ill people were identified through practice    data.

The *National Psychiatric Morbidity Survey* (Meltzer *et al.*, 1995) found a yearly prevalence rate of 4 per thousand adults, in private households, of functional psychosis (schizophrenia, manic depressive psychosis and schizo-affective disorder). This compares with a rate of 5.3 per thousand practice adult population (16 – 64) for schizophrenia and manic depression reported by the Primary Care Data Project.  The rate varied between practices from 3.1 to 6.6 per thousand. Additionally, these rates are consistent with the results produced in Liverpool, of 7.6 per 1000 practice population, and practice rates of 1.3 to 15.7 per thousand (Hoskins and Langshaw, 1995). The *National Psychiatric Morbidity Survey* used a standard interview and questionnaire for diagnosis, whereas the present study is dependent on the records of attending clinicians. However, in the majority of cases, a psychiatrist will have made the diagnoses.  The prevalence seemed to be related, on the one hand, to morbidity in the community including the presence of hostels and Care in the Community schemes; and, on the other hand, to GPs' diagnostic and treatment preferences and attitudes towards people with mental health problems. Overall, 22 (5%) people with SEMI, including 11 (8%) with schizophrenia, had no contact with their GP during the year. This compares with Liverpool, where 14 (1.6%) of people with SEMI had no contact with their GP.

The consultation rate for SEMI patients was 8.4 per person per year, similar to that found in South West Thames  (8.8 consultation per person per year), but lower that that found in Liverpool (9.4 per annum). The contact rate for this client group is much higher than that for the general population, which is 4-5 per patient per year (McCormick *et al.*, 1993), reflecting a large burden of work for primary care. Most of the

**Table 8.3 Numbers (%) of people with SEMI in contact with specialist mental health services in preceding 12 months by diagnosis**

| Diagnosis | Contact in preceding 12 months | Referred and Not seen | No contact in preceding 12 months | Not known | Total |
|---|---|---|---|---|---|
| Chronic Depression | 147(55.3) | 5(1.9) | 113(42.5) | 1(0.4) | 226(100) |
| Manic Depression | 28(75.7) | – | 9(24.3) | – | 37(100) |
| Schizophrenia | 114(83.2) | – | 22(16.1) | 1(0.7) | 137(100) |
| Total | 289(65.7) | 5(1.1) | 144(32.7) | 2(0.5) | 440(100) |

consultations were for mental health problems and minor illnesses, whereas, in a similar study in Liverpool, the majority of contacts with GPs were for mental health problems (Hoskins and Langshaw, 1995). Overall, 66% of people with SEMI were in contact with specialist mental health services, however this varied by diagnosis. Adults with psychotic diagnoses were more likely to be in contact with specialist services (83% in schizophrenia). This study did not determine levels of disability, and it is therefore not clear if the people most in need of specialist care were accessing the service.

The total Primary Care Data Project practice population of 47,212 (32,716 between 16 and 64 years old) is approximately 14% of Wirral's population. From this population, 438 people were identified with SEMI which, extrapolated to the total population of Wirral, would be approximately 3,200 patients. It will be difficult for the specialist mental health services to actively follow-up all people with SEMI. The *National Service Framework* (DoH, 1999) recognizes that, in the past, many people with SEMI lost contact with mental health services, and emphasizes the importance of the community mental health team maintaining contact. If people with SEMI are not to be lost to the mental health services, there will need to be a clear dialogue between primary and secondary care. The PCGs and PCTs will have an important role in this dialogue. The *National Service Framework* gives clear responsibility to the PCG/Ts for assessing and treating common mental health problems. NHS Trusts, however, have responsibility for people with a care programme (CPA). This will include timely access to services and follow-up in the community. It will be important that all concerned are clear who is being followed-up solely in primary care; in primary care in liaison with the specialist mental health services; and solely by the specialist mental health services. The importance of good collaboration between GPs and the specialist mental health team when caring for people with SEMI has been highlighted by other studies (King and Nazareth, 1996; Burns and Kendrick, 1997). There may be, in some instances, reluctance from those with SEMI to be followed up by specialist mental health services, as they tend to find general practice less stigmatizing (Nazareth *et al.*, 1995).

The development of care registers for people with SEMI in primary care could help in this process, provided the registers were not solely based on diagnosis but also examined how the person was coping socially and economically. The actual numbers on the register would probably be reduced considerably under these circumstances, as it is unlikely that many people with chronic depression would need to be included. The links between health and social services will also need to be clarified to ensure that registers are beneficial to this client group. A pilot project exploring the use of such registers is a subject of another chapter in this book.

## Acknowledgements

The author would like to acknowledge the contribution of Tony Kinsella, Frankanne Damato, MAAG staff, the Practice Data Analysts and all the practices involved.

## References

Burns, T. and Kendrick, T. (1997), 'Care of Long-Term Mentally Ill Patients by General Practitioners', *Psychiatric Services*, December, vol. 49, no.12, pp. 1586-8.

CHDGP Project Team (2000), *Collection of Health Data,* General Practice Guidelines, version 3, NHS Information Authority, NHSIA website (www.nhsia.nhs.uk).

Department of Health (1999), *A National Service Framework for Mental Health*, Department of Health, London.

Hoskins, A. and Langshaw, G. (1995), *Provision of Care to Practice Patients with Severe Enduring Mental Illness, Primary Care Data Project 1995*, Report for Liverpool Health Authority, Liverpool.

Kendrick, T., Burns, T., Freeling, P. and Sibbald, B. (1994), 'Provision of Care to General Practice Patients with Disabling Long-Term Illness: A Survey of 16 Practices', *British Journal of General Practice*, vol. 44, pp. 301-5.

King, M. and Nazareth, I. (1996), 'Community Care of Patients with Schizophrenia: the Role of the Primary Health Care Team', *British Journal of General Practice*, vol. 46, pp. 231-7.

McCormick, A., Fleming, D. and Charlton, J. (1993), *Morbidity Statistics from General Practice. 4th National Survey 1991-1992*, OPCS, London.

Meltzer, H., Gill, B., Petticrew, M. and Hind, K. (1995), *The Prevalence of Psychiatric Morbidity among Adults Living in Private Households. OPCS Surveys of Psychiatric Morbidity in Great Britain,* Report 1, OPCS, Series MB5, no.3, London.

Nazareth, I., King, M. and Davies, S. (1995), 'Care of Schizophrenia in General Practice: The General Practitioner and the Patient', *British Journal of General Practice*, vol. 45, pp. 343-7.

Richards, H.M., Sullivan, F.M., Mitchell, E.D. and Ross, S. (1998), 'Computer Use by General Practitioners in Scotland', *British Journal of General Practice*, vol. 48, pp. 1473-6.

Sullivan, F. and Mitchell, E. (1995), 'Has General Practitioner Computing Made a Difference to Patient Care? A Systematic Review of Published Reports', *British Medical Journal*, vol. 311, pp. 848-51.

Watkins, C., Harvey, I., Langley, C., Faulkner, A. and Gray, S. (1999), 'General Practitioners' Use of Computers During Consultation', *British Journal of General Practice*, vol. 49, pp. 381-3.

# 9 Matching Resources to Care Needs: Targeting People with Severe Mental Illness in Health and Social Services

PETER HUXLEY, SIOBHAN REILLY AND EVA ROBINSHAW

## Introduction

The project described in this chapter was designed to establish rates of severe mental illness (SMI) in both health and social services, and explore the extent to which both served similar or different populations. The research was funded as part of the Department of Health central policy research initiative. It began on January 1$^{st}$ 1997 when the mental health policy agenda was at an early stage in its present course. The data from the present study represent a unique baseline assessment of the nature of provision by community-based staff in the period immediately before the introduction of the *National Service Framework* (NSF) (DoH, 1999) and related policy. The main areas to be covered in this chapter include:

- developing a definition of SMI, which will concentrate on the 'M3' score. This is a method that conceives of SMI as a continuous rather than a categorical scale ('SMI' or 'not SMI'), which marks it out as different from other attempts at definition and allows the threshold for SMI to be varied. It also does not require a client to have a diagnosis of a psychotic illness;
- the relationship between SMI and the care programme approach (CPA) (The CPA ensures that everyone who comes to mental health services for help: has their needs assessed; is provided with a key worker; receives a care plan; and, has their needs reviewed when needed. Trusts have flexibility in deciding on what levels of CPA they chose to adopt);
- comparing health and social services;
- investigating met and unmet needs of clients with SMI characteristics; and,
- other relevant findings.

157

The authors have extensive experience in the field of mental health research. Peter Huxley founded the Mental Health Social Work Research Unit (MHSWRU) in the Department of Psychiatry at the University of Manchester in 1986. He is now Professor of Social Work at the Institute of Psychiatry in London. Both Siobhan Reilly and Eva Robinshaw work as Research Associates in the MHSWRU.

## Background

In the last decade in the UK successive governments have urged, encouraged or required health and social services to focus their attention and resources on people with SMI (House of Commons, 1990; DoH, 1993; 1994). The value and outcome of this policy are considered elsewhere in this book. This chapter is concerned with two aspects of the consequences of the policy. The first is the absence of a meaningful operational definition of SMI, and the second is the extent to which the two major staff groups providing community care to people with SMI were, in the late 1990's, already targeting their services on people with SMI.

The Mental Health Foundation (1994, p.2) recommended that the Department of Health 'promulgates a practical definition of SMI in order to concentrate attention and service on those in greatest need'. Successful targeting of resources towards people with SMI is an example of vertical target efficiency (Challis and Davies 1986), in which a high proportion of users have the appropriate characteristics for a particular service. Although the Department of Health (1995) provided some guidance about the way to define SMI, it allowed all services to arrive at their own definition. This resulted in a plethora of different definitions that risked making meaningful comparisons between services impossible. Without a standard approach it becomes difficult to compare services, sectors, or districts, in terms of the proportion of people they serve who have SMI, and hence the comparative vertical target efficiency of services remains an unknown quantity. Another consequence is a paucity of reliable health and social care data on people with SMI to inform central Government policy makers and local service delivery strategies. Information that is collected is either too broad (contract data on finished consultant episodes) or too narrow (sectioned or not). Given the duration of SMI for many people, and the need for continuous contact with services, the deficiency of detailed information impairs effective planning and monitoring of services.

The Audit Commission (1994) was the first to observe that social work caseloads had a higher proportion of SMI than nurses' caseloads. Given the policy requirement that provision for those with SMI is a priority, and the policy guidance that health and social services need to work together effectively in partnership, it is important to understand how health and social services are targeting SMI cases and how the needs of these clients are being met jointly, or otherwise, under the present arrangements.

Community psychiatric nurses (CPNs) and community based social workers (SWs) are the major staff resource in statutory services for the provision of community care. The caseloads of SWs and CPNs working in the community include many people suffering from SMI and persistent mental health problems. The current organisational arrangements mean that there are other pressures on their time, and these may reduce the focus that they are able to give to working with people with severe and persistent mental illness. For instance, many nurses in community teams have developed associations with primary care, where the demand for treatment of people without severe and persistent disorder is considerable. Many SWs in community teams are also required to provide duty services to non-mental health clients. Increasing numbers of CPNs and SWs work together in community mental health teams, frequently from the same office.

## The MARC2 (Matching Resources to Care Needs) Project

The remainder of the chapter uses data from a Department of Health funded project commissioned by the policy division. The final report of this project has been lodged with the Department of Health (Huxley *et al.*, 1999). The purpose of the project was to assess the extent to which the SMI construct could be determined by collecting empirical data on the characteristics of SMI prevalent in the literature at the time, by using a simple single page form. This was an attempt to base a definition of SMI on actual characteristics of the people receiving services, rather than an arbitrary definition based on clinical or expert judgement (see Table 9.1).

The second objective was to apply this method of assessment to the current clients of SWs and CPNs to assess the extent to which both were targeting people with these SMI characteristics. The development of the form and its reliability and validity have been described elsewhere (Huxley *et al.*, forthcoming). The data from the study represent a unique baseline assessment of the nature of provision by community-based staff in the period immediately before the introduction of the NSF and related policy measures.

## Table 9.1  Definitions of severe mental illness

<u>*Building Bridges*</u> (DoH, 1995)

Diagnosis of psychotic illness
Inability to care for themselves independently
Inability to sustain relationships
Inability to sustain work
Currently displaying florid symptoms or suffering an enduring condition
Frequent crises leading to hospital admissions
Significant risk to their own safety or that of others
Dementia; severe neurotic illness; personality disorder; developmental disorder

<u>Goldman (1981)</u>

Schizophrenia; bipolar disorder; paranoid disorder
At least one year duration
Impaired functioning in at least one of the following: occupation; family; accommodation.

<u>Tyrer *et al.*, (1995)</u>

Patients with chronic psychosis
2 or more in-patient admissions in the past year
Contact with 2 or more psychiatric agencies in the past year
Frequent consultations
Risk of imprisonment

<u>Patmore & Weaver (1990)</u>

Category A
Psychotic diagnosis, organic illness or injury
AND previous compulsory admission
OR aggregate one-year stay in hospital in past five years
OR three or more admissions in past five years
Category B
Psychotic diagnosis, organic illness or injury
OR any previous admissions in past five years
Category C
No record of hospital admissions
AND no recorded psychotic diagnosis, organic illness or injury

# Method

A cross sectional design was used to study the characteristics of clients in contact with community mental health workers in 8 locations in Britain. Six were in the North and two were in the South of England. The areas were selected to represent a range of social deprivation, and types of local authority (metropolitan borough, inner city and county areas). The community mental health staff (CPNs, SWs and occupational therapists) who were acting as a keyworker completed the MARC2 form on all of their caseload (or in some cases a random half), within a one week census period.

For some purposes, for example using multivariate statistical analyses, we have combined the pilot and main study data, giving a total sample of just over 9,500 cases. Unless specified otherwise, the results in this chapter are from the eight locations, and only for cases carried by SWs, CPNs and occupational therapists who were keyworkers (referred to in the text as the community mental health workers sample, n=3,178).

Keyworkers in these sites were also interviewed about the extent to which the client's needs were being met. For this part of the study we selected only people with a long history of care for a psychotic illness and those who were likely to remain on the worker's caseload for at least 2 months after the census period. Clients were selected randomly where numbers were sufficient and, where returns were lower, all eligible clients were selected. The study protocol envisaged obtaining a sample of 25 cases from CPNs and 25 cases from SWs in each of the eight areas, giving a total of 400 cases. Four trained researchers interviewed a total of 73 keyworkers, using a slightly adapted version of the Camberwell Assessment of Need (CAN; Phelan *et al.*, 1995) which rates a person's problem severity and degree of need in 20 areas. The MARC2 form was repeated, including the Global Assessment Scale (GAS; Endicott *et al.*, 1976) and the Health of the Nation Outcome Scales (HoNOS; Wing *et al.*, 1998). GAS is a measure of a person's level of day to day functioning at one particular point in time. HoNOS provides a profile of 12 severity ratings that can be added together to make a total score. By comparing two HoNOS scores for any person, a 'change score' - or outcome measure - can be obtained.

**Results**

*Defining Severe Mental Illness*

The scoring and items that make up each of the main definitions of SMI are varied. Patmore and Weaver's definition is made up of 2 items (for its most severe category); the *Building Bridges* definition is composed of 6 items plus diagnostic categories; Tyrer's definition has 5 items; and, Goldman's has 3 items (see Table 9.1). Instructions for interpreting and applying the definitions are limited and leave room for ambiguity.

The M3[1] score is based on a count of the 20 most heavily loaded items from a factor analysis of the total 9,500 cases (see Table 9.2). The 20 items and the method of calculation are given in the report to the Department of Health or are available from the authors. The M3 method includes a degree of flexibility in deciding where to put various thresholds, because it is made up of more items i.e. it is a continuous scale and can therefore be set to suit local circumstances. The proportion of clients having all of the defining characteristics on each of the definitions is minimal: Patmore & Weaver (3%); *Building Bridges* (zero); Tyrer (1%), Goldman (1%) and M3 (zero).

The data can be manipulated to compute a variety of definitions of SMI. Figure 9.1 shows the distribution of scores on each of the main definitions, together with scores on GAS and M3. It shows the application of three different thresholds for the M3 scores and the rates of SMI according to the different definitions, in the community mental health worker sample (n=3,178). Different proportions of the sample would be classed as SMI using the different definitions and different cut-off points. If subjects obtained two positive items (shown as 2+) on *Building Bridges*, Tyrer or M3,· then about 80% of cases would be classed as SMI. Alternatively, the Patmore & Weaver and Goldman definitions (2 items or more) would rate around 80% of the sample as having no SMI characteristics. A broad definition of SMI, like *Building Bridges*, corresponds to the lower M3 cut-off score of 2 or more items. Narrow definitions, like Patmore's and Goldman's correspond to a higher M3 cut-off score of six or more items. A cut-off point of two items on the *Building Bridges* definition produces little variation between locations (Figure 9.2).

---

[1]We are using the term M3 score to describe the overall score obtained from the MARC2 form, so that we can refer to the score and the form without confusing the two.

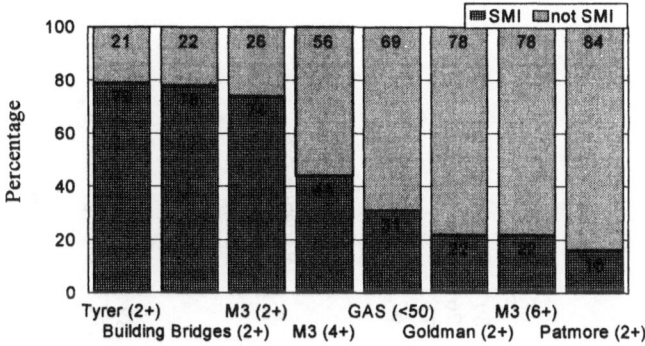

**Figure 9.1 Rates of SMI by definition**

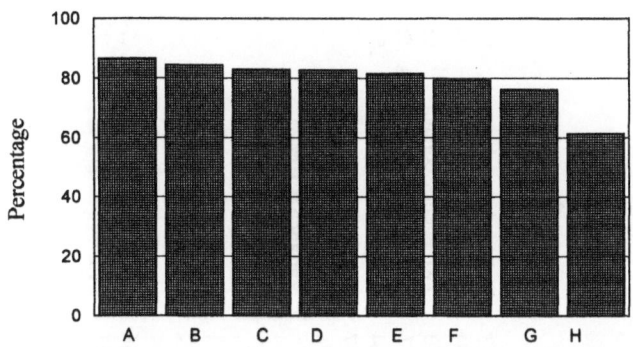

**Figure 9.2 Building Bridges – proportions scoring 2 or more items in the eight locations**

Social services' caseloads contain a higher proportion of people with the defining characteristics of SMI. Social services have a higher mean M3 score in each of the eight locations (Figure 9.3). A substantially greater proportion of the social services cases (30.2% compared to 15.4% in health; $X^2 = 86.17$, df 1, p<.001) had ever been in hospital for longer than 6 months.

**Table 9.2 Results of the factor analysis (n=9,503)**

| Factor 1 | | Factor 2 | | Factor 3 | | Factor 4 | |
|---|---|---|---|---|---|---|---|
| **Social problems** | | **Illness** | | **Aggression** | | **Suicidality** | |
| Daily occupation | .73 | Psychosis | .83 | Present (family) | .80 | Present serious | .78 |
| Relationships | .71 | Diagnosis | .78 | Present (others) | .76 | Past serious | .77 |
| Home care | .70 | Two agency contact | .63 | Past (family) | .71 | | |
| Family relations | .67 | Compulsory admissions | .58 | Past (others) | .67 | | |
| Personal care | .64 | Length of episode | .58 | | | | |
| Finances | .57 | | | | | | |
| Accommodation | .56 | | | | | | |
| Variance = 21% | | Variance = 10% | | Variance=7% | | Variance=5% | |

| Factor 5 | | Factor 6 | | Factor 7 | | Factor 8 | |
|---|---|---|---|---|---|---|---|
| **Social Exclusion** | | **Compliance** | | **Self-neglect** | | **Housing** | |
| Custody | .66 | Medication | .74 | Present | .74 | Housing | .80 |
| Substance abuse | .63 | Appointments | .72 | Past | .72 | Living situation | .61 |
| Homeless | .61 | | | | | | |
| Variance = 5% | | Variance = 4% | | Variance=4% | | Variance = 3% | |

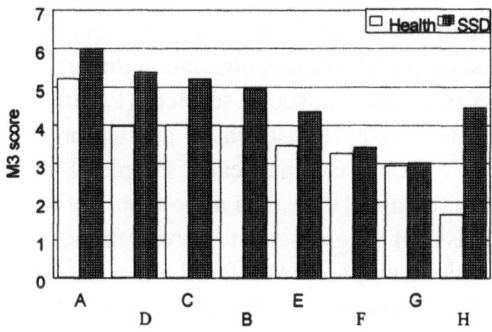

**Figure 9.3   Mean M3 scores in the eight locations**

A similar difference existed in the proportion who had ever been compulsorily admitted to hospital (50.3% in social services and 35.3% in health; $X^2 = 59.49$, df 1, p<.001).   As expected, social services have a significantly higher proportion with social problems. Those with one or more severe problems account for 51% of the social services group compared with 35% in the health group, although this latter group is dealing with greater absolute numbers of cases with moderate and severe problems (Figures 9.4 and 9.5).

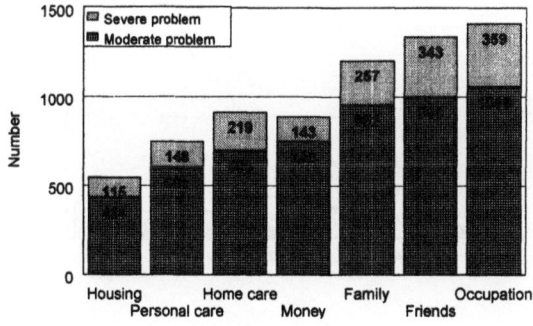

**Figure 9.4   Number of health sample (n=2,214) with social problems**

Social services cases have a greater proportion with severe current risk factors in four areas of risk (suicide, self-neglect, aggression to family and aggression to others) (Figure 9.6), and absolute numbers currently at severe risk are very similar in health and social services (Figure 9.7).

The social services sample also has a greater proportion of current moderate/severe risk factors than the health sample (Figure 9.8). In terms of absolute numbers, social services has almost half of the total cases with a moderate/severe risk of aggression towards others, 41% of those with a moderate/severe risk of aggression to family and self neglect and 36% of those with a moderate/severe risk of suicide. (Figure 9.9).

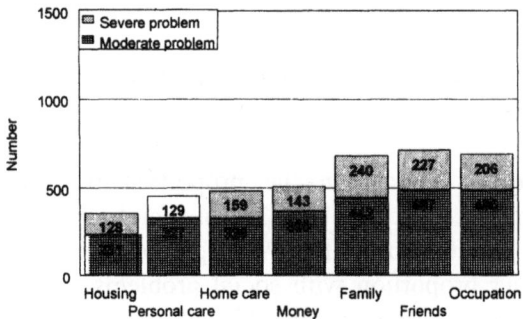

**Figure 9.5  Number of social services sample (n=964) with social problems**

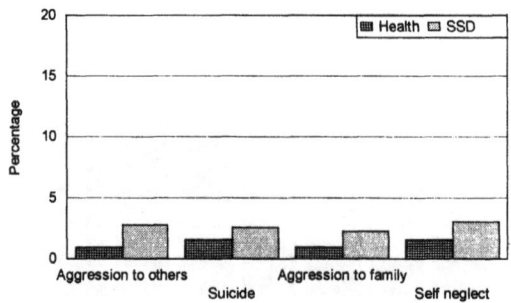

**Figure 9.6  Percentage with severe current risk factors in health and social services**

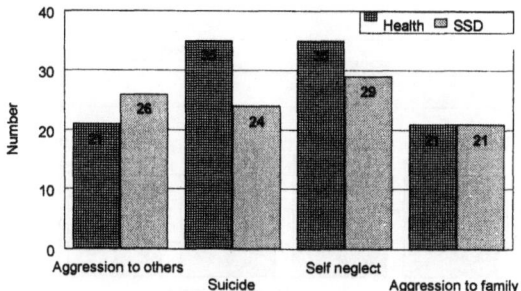

**Figure 9.7  Number with severe current risk factors in health and social services**

*Contact with Health and Social Care Services*

Cases that are dealt with by both health and social care services (n=1,539) were separated from those dealt with alone (n=1,599). The M3 scores of those dealt with jointly are significantly higher than those dealt with by a single agency (4.6 and 2.9 respectively; t = -17.7, p<.001; mean difference 1.8, 95% CI 2.0 - 1.6). This suggests that combined care is being targeted to appropriate people. Overall, social services' clients are in contact with more care agents and have a higher frequency of contact with them. However, we also found that social services' clients have more frequent contact with social care services than health care patients and vice versa. The reasons for this are not straightforward.

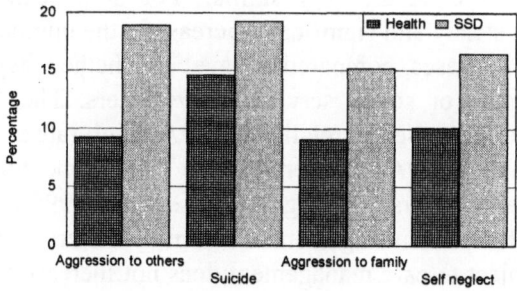

**Figure 9.8  Percentage with moderate/severe current risk factors in health and social services**

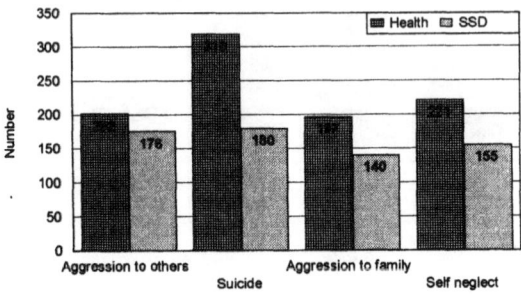

**Figure 9.9   Number with moderate/severe current risk factors in health and social services**

The findings may reflect an entirely appropriate state of affairs, with clients being referred to the correct agency in the first instance and then being allowed access, via a careful assessment process and a rational and accurate decision-making procedure, to the right forms of care to meet their needs. Thus, clients with greater social care needs receive more social care and clients with greater health care needs receive more health care. One way to throw some light on this issue, is to take the cases with the most complex mixture of health and social care needs, and see if the same still holds true. One would expect that there might be less evidence of this separation of provision in the most complex cases. One way to do this is to look separately at the cases likely to have the most complex problems, that is, those subject to the highest level of CPA and those on care management.

The results for CPA are very similar. For both health and social contacts there is a steady and significant increase in the number of contacts in a year for level 3 cases, compared to level 1, whether they were cases returned from health or social services' keyworkers. The fact that the annual contact rate increases in relation to CPA level, rather lends weight to the suggestion that CPA requirements do have some impact on this service-led picture, as others have suggested (Gilleard, 1995).

The results for care management are slightly different. In the health service, being subject to care management does not increase health service annual contacts, but does increase the number of social services contacts. In social services cases, care managed cases actually had less health service input than non-care managed cases, but had more social care contacts. In the majority of the eight study sites a greater proportion of those people that are care managed were in residential care (23% vs 6%; p<.001) and this may be one reason why they receive less health care and more social care.

Another interpretation of these results is that health and social care provision remains relatively isolated in practice, and that a service-led response remains common. It may be easier for health to make a separate healthcare provision within its own organisation, than it is to seek appropriate care elsewhere. Social services, on the other hand, will find that many clients are already in contact with the health service, but nevertheless find it easier to link the person to their network of social care provisions or contacts, than to other health care provision. This may in turn cause over provision of certain types of care/contact. Indeed, the fact that some professionals are precluded from using the resources of other agencies would exacerbate this process

One indicator of the degree of integration or separation of services is the proportion of clients who are both care managed and on CPA. This varies considerably between locations. Figure 9.10 shows a remarkable difference between the authorities in these proportions. Care management tends not to be provided without CPA. No more than 7% of clients in any of the locations are provided with care management alone. CPA on the other hand is more often provided on its own. Four of the locations provided CPA only, to over 50% of their clients.

These findings reflect very real differences in the way services are organised in each location, and this may be a suitable variable to be used as an indicator of performance, since there is great variability in it. One could argue that care management would be expected to produce a greater effect on social services' workload since it is an assessment of eligibility to receive social care services. One interpretation of these data is that CPA and care management policy are running in parallel and each is causing higher levels of provision, but the health policy causes more social provision. Greater light will be thrown on these results when the findings of the assessment of need are considered below. It may be that the needs and unmet needs of both groups of service users can be neatly divided into health and social care needs, making this pattern of provision justifiable.

One further possible explanation is that the responses of the CPNs and SWs, as well as being constrained by resource limitations, are determined by their background experience and training. Health service training predisposes one to look for and find health service solutions;

social care training predisposes one to look for and find social care solutions. Even a small amount of joint training, or the joint occupation of an office, may not influence this basic tendency. Indeed, having management and operational arrangements within the same office may even foster its continuation, through a preoccupation with the traditional division of labour.

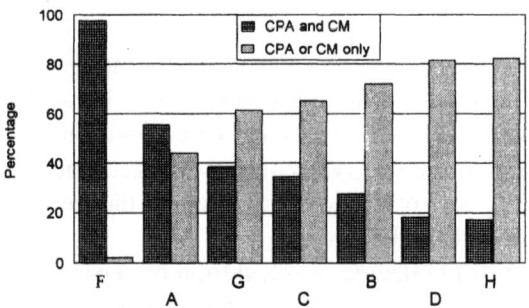

**Figure 9.10   Joint CPA and care managed clients in each location**

*Met and Unmet Needs of People with SMI Characteristics*

As well as collecting the census data, we conducted interviews with the keyworkers of randomly selected cases from the census. There were 393 interviews with keyworkers in health and social services. The results revealed no clear (or significant) difference between both agencies in the extent of client need and unmet need. The amount of unmet need and the life domains in which they occurred were remarkably similar in both agencies. Needs, therefore, cannot really be divided as suggested above.

The most common reason by far for the existence of unmet need is the client refusing to accept a service. Next comes the lack of choice, caused mainly by the inappropriate nature of some of the services on offer. These data suggest there may be an underlying disagreement about what there is a need for in many cases. This tends to confirm that the concept of need is really a negotiated construct rather than a simple objective reality.

As in the census data, those clients who had a keyworker from the health service received significantly less social service input than their counterparts who had social services' keyworkers. In contrast, the group with social services' keyworkers had a similar amount of health input as those with health keyworkers.

*Other Relevant Findings*

When compared to the national survey of new long-term in-patients (Lelliot *et al.*, 1994), this community care sample appears to have more severe problems in all areas. The individuals in the present sample who were in hospital for more than 6 months are very similar to Lelliot's new long-stay audit group; the age, gender and marital status are uncannily close. The community group has more features of severe illness and is worse off in almost every respect. This raises questions about the extent to which there is appropriate co-ordination and provision of care for these patients when they are in the community. If the community care clients are worse off than those in hospital, it is hardly surprising that they are frequently re-admitted to hospital.

A severity indicator such as M3 should change very little over time. We explored variation in the M3, GAS and HoNOS over time for cases included in the needs assessment sample. Separate ratings were made at the time the keyworkers were interviewed (on average 5 months after the census date). On the whole M3 scores changed very little over time; in contrast, the GAS and HoNOS scores change substantially over time. M3 may, therefore, be more useful for the categorization of SMI than GAS or HoNOS, which are related more to the person's current clinical state and social functioning.

Although CPNs are commonly perceived as the major provider of community care to this client group, and it is true that they are the largest group of workers in this study, there are an equal number of workers who are not CPNs. When all workers are included, CPNs make up 48% of the total.

## Conclusion

When considering the issue of the absence of a meaningful operational definition of SMI, it is clear that the M3 method includes a degree of flexibility that the other definitions do not have. This is important in various areas. It enables purchasers and research staff to compare services, agencies and programmes by using a consistent set of items that can be completed easily by professional staff, and it can be used to assess the extent to which services and programmes are targeting on people with similar profiles.

The study revealed a difference in the proportion of cases having the characteristics associated with SMI, in health and social services. Social services' cases have a greater proportion of SMI characteristics and, in some risk categories, similar numbers of clients at current risk as do health services. So far as targeting SMI is concerned, this shows that the social services caseloads were better targeted than the caseloads of community health staff.

Social services' cases have more contact with social care services (and equal contact with health care services) but there is no difference in the extent of met and unmet need between the two groups. There was no clear tendency for health to produce superior outcomes on HoNOS health items, nor for social services to produce superior outcomes on the HoNOS social items. So, although considerable numbers of people with SMI were targeted to receive services, the logic of providing them separately in health and social services received no support in the present study. The results therefore raise serious questions about the benefits of providing health and social care services separately to this client group.

# References

Audit Commission (1994), *Finding A Place: A Review of Mental Health Services for Adults*, HMSO, London.

Challis, D. and Davies, B. (1986), *Case Management in Community Care*, Gower, Aldershot.

Department of the Environment, Transport and the Regions (1998), *1998 Index of Local Deprivation*, HMSO, London.

Department of Health (1993), *The Health of the Nation*, HMSO, London.

Department of Health (1994), *The Key Area Handbook – Mental Illness*, 2nd Edition, HMSO, London.

Department of Health (1995), *The Health of the Nation. Building Bridges: A Guide to Arrangements for Inter-Agency Working for the Care and Protection of Severely Mentally Ill People*, HMSO, London.

Department of Health (1998), *Partnerships in Action (New Opportunities for Joint Working between Health and Social Services): A Discussion Document*, HMSO, London.

Department of Health (1999), *A National Service Framework for Mental Health*, Department of Health, London.

Endicott, J., Spitzer, R.L., Fleiss, J.L. and Cohen, J. (1976), 'The Global Assessment Scale', *Archives of General Psychiatry*, vol. 33, pp. 766-71.

Gilleard, C. (1995), 'Implementation of the Care Programme Approach in the Community', *Psychiatric Bulletin*, vol. 19, no. 12, pp. 750-2.

Goldman, H. (1981), 'Defining and Counting the Chronically Mentally Ill', *Hospital and Community Psychiatry*, vol. 32, pp. 21-2.

Harrison, J., Barrow, S. and Creed, F. (1995), 'Social Deprivation and Psychiatric Admission Rates among Different Diagnostic Groups', *British Journal of Psychiatry*, vol. 167, pp. 456-62.

House of Commons (1990), *The NHS and Community Care Act*, HMSO, London.

Huxley, P.J., Reilly, S. and Robinshaw, E. (1999), *The Care Provided by Health and Social Services to People with the Characteristics of Severe Mental Illness*, Final Report to the Department of Health, School of Psychiatry, University of Manchester, Manchester.

Huxley, P.J., Reilly, S. and Robinshaw, E. (2000), *Matching Resources to Care: The Acceptability, Validity and Inter-Rater Reliability of a New Instrument to Assess Severe Mental Illness (MARC-1)*, forthcoming.

Lelliot, P., Wing, J. and Clifford, P. (1994), 'A National Audit of New Long-Stay Psychiatric Patients I: Method and Description of the Cohort', *British Journal of Psychiatry*, vol. 165, pp. 160-9.

Mental Health Foundation (1994), *Creating Community Care*, Mental Health Foundation, London.

Patmore, C. and Weaver, J. (1990), *A Survey of Community Mental Health Centres*, Good Practices in Mental Health, London.

Phelan, M., Slade, M., Thornicroft, G., Dunn, G., Holloway, F., Wykes, T., Strathdee, G., Loftus, L., McCrone, P. and Hayward, P. (1995), 'The Camberwell Assessment of Need: The Validity and Reliability of an Instrument to Assess the Needs of People with Severe Mental Illness', *British Journal of Psychiatry*, vol. 167, pp. 589-95.

Tyrer, P., Turner, R. and Johnson, A.L. (1989), 'Integrated Use of Hospital and Community Psychiatric services and Use of In-Patient Beds', *British Medical Journal*, vol. 299, pp. 298-300.

Tyrer, P., Morgan, J., Van-Horn, E., Jayakody, M., Evans, K., Brummell, R., White, T., Baldwin, D., Harrison-Read, P. and Johnson, T. (1995), 'A Randomised Controlled Study of Close Monitoring of Vulnerable Psychiatric Patients', *Lancet*, vol. 345, no. 8952, pp. 756-9.

Wing, J.K., Beevor, A.S., Curtis, R.H., Park, S.B.G., Hadden, S. and Burns, A. (1998), 'Health of the Nation Outcomes Scales: Research and Development', *British Journal of Psychiatry*, vol. 172, pp. 11-18.

# 10 Mental Health Registers in Primary Care: A Case Study in Service Targeting

WALLY BARR AND LESLEY COTTERILL

## Introduction

In order to target mental health services on those with the greatest needs, it is of fundamental importance that these individuals can be readily identified. One initiative which may facilitate this is the development of mental health registers, held in general practices, which contain the names of all practice patients with a severe and enduring mental illness (SEMI). This chapter will describe a research project which has evaluated one such initiative in an English health district. This three-year study, which reported in May 2000, was developed specifically to monitor the process, and evaluate the impact on patients and carers, of introducing primary care-held SEMI registers into a range of general practices. It was funded by the NHS Executive (North West Regional Office) Research and Development Directorate. The chapter begins with a resume of the history and principles underlying the introduction of SEMI registers into primary care. It then describes the background to the present study and the methods employed. Some preliminary findings are presented and their implications for practice and future research are discussed.

The authors have been involved in a range of social research studies in the fields of community care and mental health. Wally Barr is currently a research fellow in the Health and Community Care Research Unit (HaCCRU), University of Liverpool. Lesley Cotterill previously worked in HaCCRU and the Oxford Centre for Health Care Research and Development. She is now a freelance researcher.

## Primary Care-Held SEMI Registers

The *National Service Framework for Mental Health* (DoH, 1999) makes it clear that it is essential for specialist mental health services to retain contact with people who have severe and enduring mental illness, especially those presenting a risk to themselves or others. In order that specialist mental health providers do not become overwhelmed by the sheer volume of referrals they receive, it is important that GPs and others are able to decide which patients are most appropriate for referral to specialist care. Similarly, the capacity of mental health specialists to filter referrals they receive through a mechanism that readily and consistently identifies those who meet their acceptance criteria, is a pre-requisite to them targeting services on their primary concern: patients with a severe and enduring mental illness. Operationally, this system depends on a commonly agreed and precise definition of the term 'severe and enduring mental illness'. Despite the importance of this, there is little agreement over the dimensions or thresholds which should be used to identify this priority group (Barr and Cotterill, 1999a; Slade *et al.*, 1997). This is of crucial importance, since the collection of names and details of all those who fulfil specific service-entry criteria is an essential ingredient in the development of a needs-led mental health service (Kingdon, 1996; Slade *et al.*, 1997).

Psychiatric registers offer considerable potential to facilitate service targeting once basic service-entry criteria have been established. They can be held within either the primary or secondary care sectors, yet it is only in recent years that they have come to be used to assist in focusing services on specifically defined and vulnerable groups. The register of SEMI patients in the Paddington area of London, for example, was set up in 1990 (Tyrer *et al.*, 1995) in order to target those with either a psychotic illness, wide or prolonged usage of psychiatric services or frequent psychiatric in-patient admission. On a national scale, the introduction of Supervision Registers in 1994 represents a clear example of the use of registers to facilitate service targeting. These registers contain details of only those people with SEMI who have been deemed to represent a significant risk to either themselves or others (DoH, 1994a) and, as with previous psychiatric case registers, these are kept by local specialist provider units.

In many ways, the introduction of Supervision Registers set the scene for the general establishment of care registers of those people with SEMI. The siting of psychiatric registers has virtually always rested with the provider agencies responsible for *secondary* specialist care. It has been pointed out that the presence of SEMI registers in *primary* care has been relatively rare (Kendrick *et al.*, 1991), although there has subsequently been a small amount of research into the establishment of mental health registers in general practice (Kendrick *et al.*, 1994). Another research study into the provision of care to SEMI patients has made the recommendation that primary health care teams should be enabled to develop care registers (Hoskins and Langshaw, 1996). These researchers concluded that inclusion on the registers should be based on disability as well as diagnosis and it was anticipated that registers would allow those working in both primary and secondary care settings to clarify their roles in respect of each registered patient. Registers were also expected to allow the amount of support provided by community mental health teams (CMHTs) to primary health care teams (PHCTs), to be based on morbidity levels in their practice populations as well as on levels of expertise within the PHCTs themselves (*ibid*).

The introduction of practice-based SEMI registers may have a number of unintended consequences, including the further stigmatization of registered patients and professional concerns about increased clinical responsibility (Barr and Cotterill, 1999b). Nevertheless, in practical terms, it has been demonstrated that the establishment of SEMI registers is quite feasible in relatively well organised and computerised general practices (Nazareth *et al.*, 1993a). This can be achieved largely through the use of diagnostic entries and prescription histories, involving the identification of patients in receipt of psychotropic medication (*ibid*). However, it should be remembered that a small number of SEMI patients do not consult over a period of years and may be unknown to their GP (Goldberg and Jackson, 1992; Hassall and Stilwell, 1977; Kendrick *et al.*, 1994). These patients will clearly fail to be registered and, therefore, will continue to represent a source of some concern.

## Background to the Present Study

The research study described here commenced in May 1997 and finally reported in May 2000. It was conducted in an English health district where registers were being compiled in each general practice, listing details of all practice patients with severe and enduring mental illness. Throughout the period when registers were being set up, the district was undergoing considerable internal restructuring, involving the merger of two NHS trusts and establishment of three multi-disciplinary CMHTs to provide community mental health services.

The registers were drawn up by community mental health nurses (CPNs), who were each based within the newly established CMHTs, whilst also being linked to specific general practices across the district. These

CPNs were advised by their management to liaise extensively with practice GPs and other primary care staff in order to ensure the accuracy of registers. Criteria for inclusion on the registers were based on the definition of 'severe and enduring mental illness' which has been offered by the Department of Health (DoH, 1995a). This centres on the dimensions of safety, informal/formal care, diagnosis, disability and duration of illness. The registers were compiled from the patient population of each general practice rather than solely from the caseloads of secondary service providers. They therefore should include the very significant proportion of individuals with severe mental illness who rely entirely on their GP for medical care and long-term psychotropic medication and who have no contact with secondary specialist services (Kendrick *et al., 1994*).

**Aims of the study**

The general aims of the study were to *monitor* the process of establishing SEMI registers in primary care settings and to *evaluate* whether registers made a difference to the quality of care and quality of life of patients and carers. The specific hypotheses under examination in the evaluative element of the study were that registers would facilitate improvements in:

- patients' levels of need for help from a range of statutory services;
- patients' quality of life (QOL);
- carers' experiences; and,
- the co-ordination and use of mental health services.

**Methods**

The research design was action-oriented so the study could be responsive to changes in the implementation of the 'Registers Initiative' and results be disseminated as soon as practicable. There were over 60 general practices in the district under scrutiny and by the autumn of 1997 SEMI registers had begun to be established in almost all of these. Throughout the following year these registers were subject to a process of refinement, by the link CPNs and practice GPs, with the intention that they should contain all practice patients with a severe and enduring mental illness.

*Selection of Sample Practices*

We wished to select a small number of general practices which were representative of all practices within the district. Practices throughout the district were known to be sited in areas of widely varying affluence and social deprivation (Sykes and Smith, 1995). However, the fact that the 6 original health locality boundaries in the district were based on socio-economic parameters provided a basis for the selection of sample practices. Firstly, 6 practices were randomly selected from within each of the 6 localities. Partners in each of these 36 practices were approached by letter with details of the study and invited to take part. A total of 17 practices expressed a willingness to participate and each practice was then visited by WB to discuss the implications of this. From these 17 practices, which were reasonably well distributed across the 6 health localities, one from each locality was randomly selected to participate in the study.

*Monitoring the Process of Establishing SEMI Registers*

The method used to monitor the introduction of the registers was a series of semi-structured interviews. These were conducted with those members of staff who had made the greatest input into establishing the SEMI registers in the six sample practices. These 'key informants' consisted of the six link CPNs along with the practice managers and interested GPs from the participating practices. They were interviewed individually on three separate occasions – in the autumns of 1997 and 1998 and in the summer of 1999 – which generated data concerning experiences of setting-up and refining the registers. Although not transcribed, all interviews were audiotaped. They comprised of a confidential discussion with each key informant based on a topic list which had been generated during a prior series of piloting interviews with others who had been involved in setting-up similar registers.

*Evaluating the Impact of Registers on Patients and Carers.*

Service usage and demographic data relating to all patients on the registers of the six sample practices (the 'basic patient sample') were compared over the years 1997, 1998 and 1999. As part of this quantitative evaluation, a sub-sample of patients was drawn from the basic patient sample which allowed a more detailed examination of the effects of registration on patient functioning. These patients, including (where appropriate) their carers, were interviewed on two occasions: at baseline during the period April to October 1998 (before the registers could have had a significant impact) and at follow-up approximately 12 months later.

*Selection of patient sub-sample* Patients' names were randomly selected from the SEMI registers of the sample practices. This process was stratified to ensure the sample was representative in terms of gender, diagnosis and age. Following agreement from the local Health Research Ethics Committee, selected patients were contacted by the manager of their general practice with information about the study and were offered a date for interview with the researchers. A pre-printed letter and stamped envelope addressed to the researchers were included for return by any patient not wishing to participate in the research. All consenting patients were visited and interviewed by WB, and recruitment to the patient sub-sample was brought to a close at the end of October 1998.

*Selection of carer sample* In order to generate data concerning the impact of SEMI registers on carers, their experiences were assessed during visits to conduct the patient interviews. Each patient from the sub-sample was invited to nominate one friend or relative whom they defined to be providing some degree of care, and each carer was asked to complete a questionnaire relating to their personal perceptions of this role.

*Instruments* The patient characteristics most likely to be responsive to the improved care which registers could facilitate, were felt to be 'need' in a broad sense, and quality of life. Two questionnaires which would generate this data, were therefore applied during interviews with each member of the sub-sample, between April and October 1998. The particular instruments – the *Camberwell Assessment of Need* (CAN) (Phelan *et al.*, 1995) and the *Life Fulfilment Scale* (LFS) (Baker *et al.*, 1994) – have both been found to have reliable and valid properties. The CAN (research version 3.0) assesses levels of clinical and social need in 22 domains. It allows both the patient and their keyworker to provide independent ratings, but in the present study only patient ratings were used because relatively few subjects were found to have specialist mental health keyworkers. The LFS operationalises life fulfilment in terms of the discrepancy between respondents' desired and actual circumstances. It was used during the personal interviews with each subject in the sub-sample, following administration of the CAN. The LFS consists of 13 items, or life domains, and a fulfilment score is generated in each of these. The instrument used to gather data concerning carers' experiences, the *Experience of Caregiving Inventory* (ECI) (Szmukler *et al.*, 1996a), was designed specifically for use by a relative or friend caring for someone with a serious mental illness.

*Data Analysis*

*Monitoring the introduction of registers* Audiotaped interview data were thematically analysed to draw out commonalties and differences between respondents. Because data were gathered on three occasions over a period of two years, changing experiences over time could be identified.

*Evaluating the effects of registers on patients and carers* Needs for services and quality of life of patients in the sub-sample, were compared between the baseline and follow-up assessments. The paired t-test and McNemar test (using the binomial distribution where expected frequencies were small) were applied to these paired data. The chi-square test was adopted to analyse data relating to contact with mental health services at baseline. All tests were two-tailed and statistical probability was set at the customary level of $p = 0.05$. All statistical analysis was carried out using *SPSS for Windows*, version 9.0.

## Results

Results reported in this chapter are based on a preliminary analysis of the research data.[1]

*Monitoring the Process of Establishing SEMI Registers.*

Initial discussions and interviews with a range of stakeholders in the sample practices (practice managers, link CPNs and GPs) generated considerable data. Analysis of these data is reported here under the main themes to emerge: *defining 'SEMI'*; *setting-up a SEMI register*; *problems encountered*; and, *the implications of registers.*

*Defining 'SEMI'* Although all link CPNs had based the registers on the definition offered in the Department of Health report *Building Bridges* (DoH, 1995a), it was clear that this definition is rather broad and open to

---

[1] At the time of going to press, data analysis was ongoing.

interpretation in a number of ways. During the course of the interviews, all informants expressed the view that patients suffering from a psychotic illness should be included within the definition of SEMI, as well as patients with on-going needs who required support from services over a period of time. The actual time period specified by informants in relation to the notion of 'enduring' mental illness varied from 6 months to 2 years, and generally related to the use of secondary mental health services. However, all informants agreed that patients with non-psychotic diagnoses could readily belong to this category. Such patients would be likely to suffer from some form of depression, although some informants mentioned other disabling conditions, such as severe anxiety, including phobic reactions and obsessional/compulsive disorders. Only one informant directly referred to the possibility of including the notion of 'disability' in the definition of SEMI.

It was clear that informants did not share a specific definition of SEMI. There was some confusion as to whether the diagnosis of *anxiety* should ever be included, even when severe and, as mentioned, conceptions of 'enduring' varied considerably. Only one informant actually specified the long-term use of primary care services for mental health care as constituting an 'enduring' disorder in the absence of use of any secondary specialist mental health services.

*Setting-up a SEMI register*   The initial composition of the SEMI registers in the six sample practices varied considerably in terms of patient diagnosis and prevalence of SEMI in practice populations. This was particularly evident in the two main diagnostic groupings, schizophrenia (n=69) and depression (n=128), as shown in Figure 10.1. Some refinement was made over subsequent months, but there remained little sign that the registers had been used proactively, as working tools which could inform practice within primary care teams. The process of drawing-up the registers initially involved a number of approaches common to all sample practices. Firstly, a computerised search was made of CPN current and past caseloads for patients who met the SEMI definition.[2] A similar search was made of recent in-patient admissions to the local psychiatric hospital, as well as patients currently seeing a hospital psychiatrist as an outpatient. The second stage involved CPNs providing their link practice GPs with a list of anti-psychotic medications, and requesting that the practice database be searched to generate the names of patients in receipt of any of these. All but

---

[2] NB: the time period of the search varied between informants.

two of the CPN informants highlighted the fact that they, or practice GPs, had removed the names of patients where the dosage of medication suggested a non-psychotic diagnosis (e.g. chlorpromazine when prescribed in low doses as an anti-emetic and thioridazine when given in low doses as an anxiolytic). In the third stage, the CPN lists and practice lists were combined by the CPN and the resulting list was sometimes, but not always, discussed with primary health care team staff, including GPs, before being presented as the practice SEMI register.

So far as we could ascertain, in only one practice had primary health care staff conducted a systematic examination of the register after receiving it from the CPN. In this particular practice, GPs were asked to examine the register and to remove the names of any patients inappropriately included. Informants reported that in none of the sample practices were the registers held in computerised form; in all six practices the register existed only in the form of a typed list of names kept in a folder. The only other copy of the registers was kept in the CMHT office (i.e. the base of the relevant 'link CPN'). This has implications for confidentiality and access to registers, as well as the likelihood of the register being used as an active resource. Informants were unaware of any system for updating the information on registers and some diversity of opinion was apparent as to where responsibility for the task of updating/reviewing registers, should lie. Whereas some felt the GP should update the register, others felt the CPN would be expected to do this. Nevertheless, most stressed the need for improved liaison between CPNs and GPs if registers were to reflect an accurate and up-to-date picture.

*Problems encountered in setting-up registers* Problems encountered by those who had drawn-up registers, particularly the link CPNs, varied a little, but there were commonalties in their experiences:

- Firstly, almost all CPN informants identified constraints of time as an important issue. The process of identifying SEMI patients was seen by a number of informants as an extra task in an already busy job. It should perhaps be noted that CPNs were asked to compile registers at a time of widespread organisational change, including the merger of the local Community NHS Trust with a neighbouring Trust, and planning discussions to establish multidisciplinary CMHTs across the district.

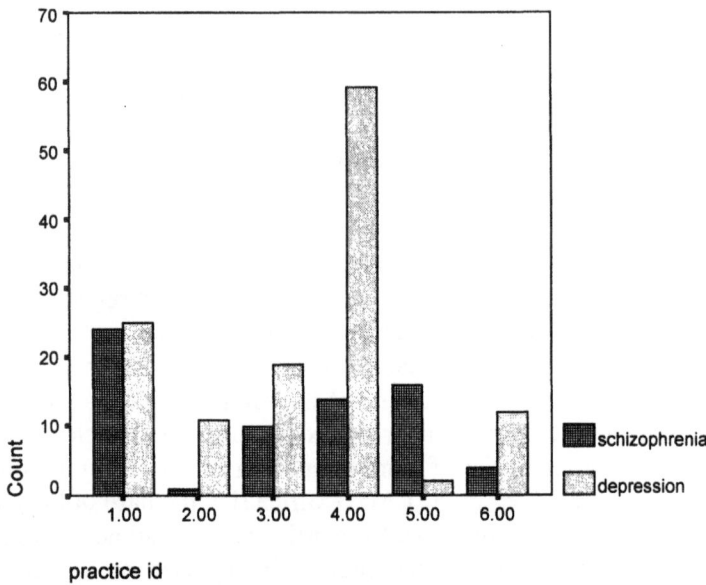

**Figure 10.1    Sample practice registers at baseline assessment: patients with schizophrenia or depression**

- Secondly, the vagueness of the definition of 'SEMI' was highlighted by some informants as a further potential source of difficulty.
- Thirdly, an area of difficulty identified by most informants was a need for clarification on the part of GPs concerning the reasoning behind, and the implications of, the introduction of SEMI registers. Whilst a certain amount of GP resistance was anecdotally reported in isolated examples, no informant expressed the opinion that this had been a problem within the six sample practices. On the other hand, informants gave the impression that they themselves were unsure of the reasoning behind the introduction of registers and we therefore presume they would have been in a poor position to reassure or to inform GPs.

Essentially, informants found the task of establishing the registers to be somewhat tedious. There was an absence of protocols from the Trust to guide this process, but most of the informants were unable to identify any specific factor that would have significantly eased the task. Only one respondent ventured the suggestion that a fully computerised information system might have allowed ready access to patient details without the need to consult documents held on files.

*Implications of registers*  Informants from all professional backgrounds were unanimous in expressing the view that patients will not know that their names have been included on a SEMI register. Views as to whether patients should have a right to know this were somewhat varied, with most informants recognising the potentially stigmatising nature of registration. Problems with access to, and security of, registers were recognised by some informants who compared them with other registers, such as primary care-held diabetes and asthma registers, and social services child-at-risk registers. There was ultimately considerable variation among informants concerning the balance between the rights of a patient to have their name removed from a register at their request, and the need to find systems which will identify people who may lack insight and may not be receiving the services they need.

Informants' views concerning the introduction of SEMI registers ranged from the optimistic to the distinctly pessimistic. One felt, for example, that the introduction of registers would strengthen the position of CPNs in rejecting inappropriate referrals, such as those patients who would not be eligible for registration. Another pointed out that registers have the potential for identifying needy patients unknown to the specialist services. However, on the pessimistic side, one informant ventured the opinion that registers are unlikely to have any great impact, since CPNs already know the client group and, therefore, don't need registers, while GPs are unlikely to use them anyway.

Informants were agreed, by the summer of 1999, that registers had made little impact and were not yet working documents. Only one informant expressed the view that registers would be unlikely to ever have a positive impact on patient care. A more optimistic tone was detected in others, with one informant pointing out that, if nothing else, registers have clarified the main target group for CPNs, and although GP's may not agree with this policy change, registers have played a part in focusing their attention on SEMI patients. Nevertheless, several CPN informants made the observation that they continued to receive 'inappropriate' referrals from GPs. Whether the introduction of SEMI registers would improve this was seen as unlikely, given the current inadequacy of primary care based counselling services to meet the needs of patients with less severe mental health problems. Only one informant recognised the potential of registers to highlight the differential workloads of general practices across the district. This aspect of SEMI registers is important for service planning, since it has implications for the allocation of CPN time to practices.

## Evaluating the Impact of Registers on Patients and Carers

Within the six sample practices, patient populations ranged from over 2,800 to nearly 12,000, with one practice having only 2 partners and others as many as 6 (see Table 10.1). Numbers of patients on the sample SEMI registers totalled 274 at the end of baseline data collection on 31st October 1998.

### Basic Patient Sample

*Demography* The mean age of the 274 patients included on the registers was 45 years (sd=12 years). Ninety-three subjects were aged under forty, and 181 were aged forty or more. The majority of subjects were female (n=147, males n=127), and primary diagnoses included depression (n=128); schizophrenia (n=69); anxiety (n=32); bi-polar affective disorder (n=27); schizo-affective disorder (n=3); and, personality disorder (n=1). Data on the diagnostic details of 14 subjects were unclear from their primary care notes.

*Use of mental health services* In the final months of 1998, link CPNs and practice GPs were expected to continue the process of refining their SEMI registers to ensure they accurately reflected the practice population in terms of patients with SEMI characteristics. In the six sample practices, the number of patients on the registers totalled 253 at the end of December 1998. This represented a reduction from the 274 in October and was due to a refinement of some of the registers. Preliminary data analysis revealed that 101 of these 253 patients were in contact with specialist mental health services at 31st December 1998 (this included contact with psychiatrists, psychologists, CPNs, mental health social workers or mental health support workers based in CMHTs). When the demographic characteristics of those subjects in, or not in, contact with mental health services were compared, they were found to differ significantly in respect of only two factors.

**Table 10.1 Practices by size, number of partners and size of SEMI register at baseline assessment**

| Practice | 1* | 2* | 3* | 4* | 5 | 6* | Total |
|---|---|---|---|---|---|---|---|
| Approx. list size | 7,500 | 4,500 | 9,100 | 12,000 | 4,800 | 2,800 | 40,700 |
| Number of partners | 5 | 3 | 5 | 6 | 3 | 2 | 24 |
| Number of patients on SEMI register | 66 | 14 | 38 | 98 | 33 | 25 | 274 |

* originally fundholding practices

Firstly, subjects varied in their practice affiliation: in two of the six sample practices, less than one quarter of patients were in specialist contact, whereas the position was reversed in two of the other practices ($X^2 = 77.58$; df=5; p<.001). The second finding was within diagnostic groupings: while numbers of subjects with schizophrenia were fairly evenly divided in terms of service contact (with 30 being in contact, and 35 not in contact with mental health services), subjects with depression were significantly less likely to be in contact with these specialist services than all other diagnostic groups ($X^2 = 5.31$; df=1; p=.03). In all, less than one third of the 158 subjects with a neurotic diagnosis were in contact with mental health services, whereas over half the 95 subjects with a psychotic diagnosis had specialist contact ($X^2 = 8.62$; df=1; p=.003).

## Patient Sub-Sample

From the basic sample of all patients on the six sample registers (n=274) a total of 135 patient names were randomly selected. Contact was made with 128 of these individuals, seven being excluded from contact at the request of their GP because of their perceived inability to provide considered responses to researchers' questions. Of the 128 contacted patients, we received no response from 37, the reasons for this being unknown. From the group of 91 who did respond, 42 declined participation in the study, again for reasons unknown, and 49 agreed. The chi-square test revealed no significant differences between these two latter groups in terms of their known demographic variables – age, gender, primary diagnosis and practice affiliation. The sub-sample, therefore, consisted of 49 patients, who were fairly evenly split in terms of gender (males: n= 25; females: n=24) and diagnosis (psychosis: n = 28; neurosis: n = 21), which was consistent with the stratified sampling approach adopted for the study. At baseline, less than half the subjects in the sub-sample (37%) lived alone, and only six (12%) were in any form of paid employment. Whilst only two subjects lived in 24-hour residential care, 13 (27%) by their own definition, were to some extent provided with care by others. At the follow-up assessment 12 months later, 40 of the original sub-sample of 49 subjects were re-interviewed and assessed using the CAN, LFS and ECI for carers. Three of those not seen declined a repeat interview, three could not be contacted, two were unable to complete the interview and one subject had died.

*Extent of need in the patient sub-sample* Findings reported in this section relate only to those subjects who were assessed at both baseline and follow-up. As illustrated in Figure 10.2, 'need' (whether met or not) was found to exist in the greatest number of subjects at each assessment episode in the domains of *psychological distress, daytime activities,* and *physical health.* Conversely, the domains where the least number of subjects expressed need were *safety to others* and *drugs.* The pattern of needs set at baseline remained substantially unchanged 12 months later at the follow-up assessment, since none of the 22 CAN domains was found to have changed significantly (McNemar/binomial test).

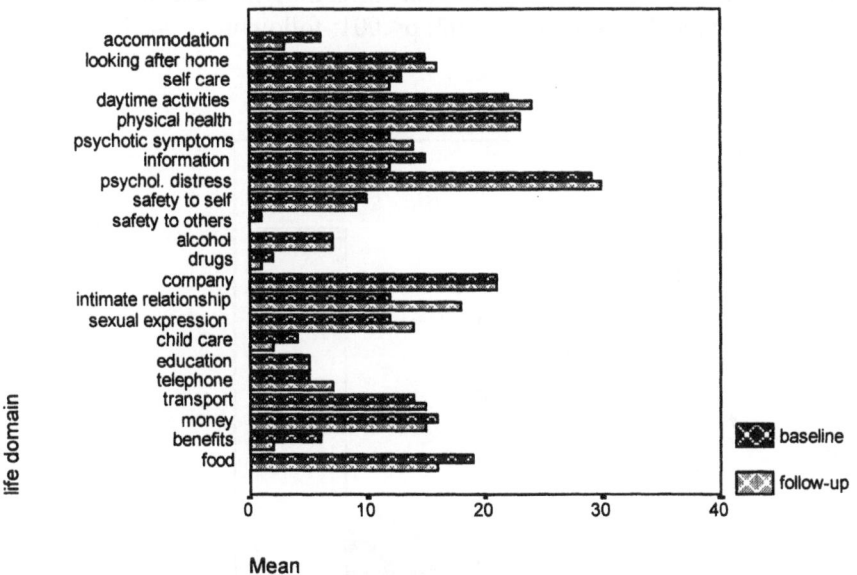

**Figure 10.2** **Numbers of subjects with need at baseline and follow-up assessments**

Table 10.2 shows the results of a comparison between the *overall* need at both the baseline and follow-up assessments. The first row of the table – *number of needs* – indicates the mean number of domains in which subjects had needs at baseline and follow-up to have been 7.22 and 7.08 respectively (out of a possible maximum of 22) – a non-significant result (paired t-test: t=0.25; p=.80). The next row – *level of needs* – similarly shows no significant change over time. The final two rows in Table 10.2 illustrate the *levels of help needed and given* by local (formal) agencies, such as the statutory social and health services. Neither the *level of formal help needed,* nor the *level given,* was found to have significantly changed in the 12 months between baseline and follow-up assessments.

*Unmet need* When the mean *level of formal help needed* is compared with the mean *level of formal help given,* a measure of unmet need is generated (Slade *et al.*, 1994). Paired t-tests revealed that, in those for whom full data were available, there was a significant difference in these scores at each assessment episode (baseline: t=6.02; p<.001; follow-up: t=4.57; p<.001) – see Figure 10.3.

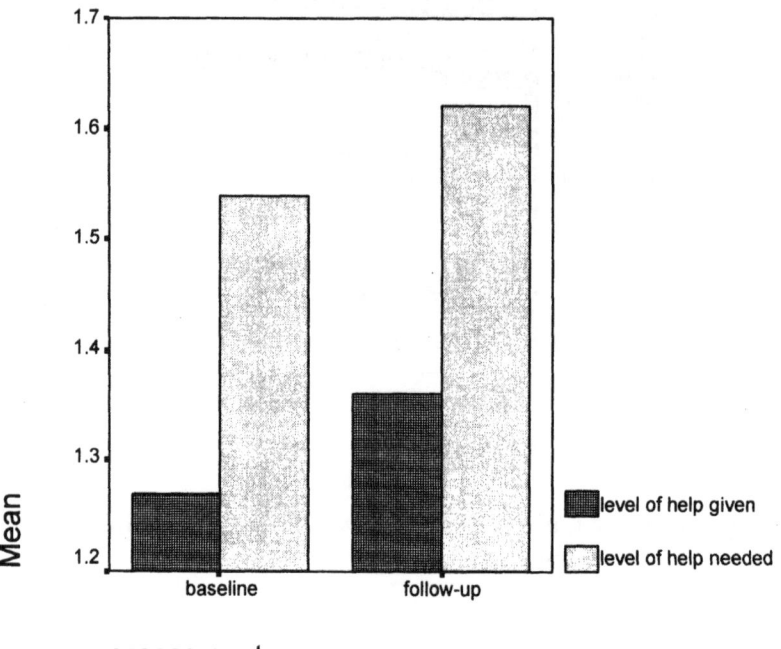

**Figure 10.3    Levels of help given and needed from local (formal) services at baseline and follow-up assessment**

**Table 10.2 Comparison of the extent of need and unmet need for help from local services at baseline and follow-up assessments**

| | n[1] | Baseline Mean (sd) | Follow-up Mean (sd) | t value[2] | P value |
|---|---|---|---|---|---|
| Number of needs | 37 | 7.22 (3.43) | 7.08 (3.58) | 0.25 | 0.80 |
| Level of needs | 37 | 9.35 (4.57) | 9.14 (5.24) | 0.25 | 0.80 |
| Level of formal help needed | 36 | 1.53 (0.46) | 1.60 (0.42) | -0.82 | 0.41 |
| Level of formal help given | 33 | 1.31. (0.49) | 1.38 (0.42) | -0.84 | 0.42 |

1. Based on subjects who were assessed at both baseline and follow-up    2. Paired t-tests; all tests 2-tailed

This finding indicates that the significant *level of unmet need for formal services* that existed in the sample at baseline assessment, effectively remained 12 months later at the follow-up assessment. This was the case despite the introduction of SEMI registers, which theoretically had the potential to facilitate a more appropriate targeting of services and so to reduce levels of unmet need by the follow-up assessment.

Nevertheless, bivariate correlations for *formal help needed* and *formal help given* at both assessment episodes, showed them to be strongly and positively correlated on each occasion (baseline: r=0.78; p<.001; follow-up: r=0.64; p<.001). This means that those subjects with the greatest levels of need were in receipt of the greatest levels of help from local services. To some extent this can be taken as an indication that service targeting was at least moderately effective at both assessment points. Nevertheless, the high levels of unmet need show that, although those with the greatest need received the greatest amount of help, the level of help they received failed to fully meet their needs.

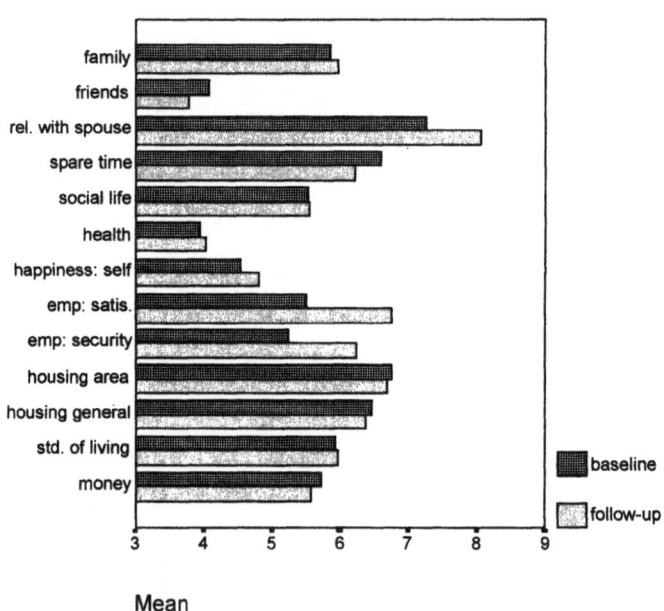

Mean

**Figure 10.4  Life fulfilment ratings at baseline and follow-up assessment**

those subjects who were assessed on each occasion. Greatest fulfilment was found to lie in the domain *relationship with spouse*; the domains attracting the lowest ratings of fulfilment were those of *health* and *having close friends*. It is again apparent that the pattern established at baseline remained effectively unchanged at follow-up. This was confirmed by the paired t-test, which showed no significant changes to have taken place in any of the 13 LFS domains.

Moderately strong and significant correlations were also found in several domains: *fulfilment with health* at baseline and follow-up assessments ($r=0.67$; $p<.001$); *money* ($r=0.57$; $p<.001$); *social life* ($r=0.59$; $p<.001$) and *standard of living* ($r=0.50$; $p=.002$). These results further indicate that subjects' levels of fulfilment in these particular areas of life have remained essentially unchanged over time.

*Carers' Experiences*

The 66 items in the ECI are grouped into 10 scales. Results have been adjusted to their original scoring (which indicated the frequency with which specific thoughts came to mind: 0='never'; 1='rarely'; 2='sometimes'; 3='often', and 4='nearly always'). This facilitates comparison between scales. Nevertheless, interpretation of the results has been hampered by the small numbers of people in the analysis: at the baseline assessment only 11 carers completed an ECI questionnaire. At follow-up this number fell to 10 and of these, only six carers had completed questionnaires at both assessment episodes. Statistical analysis was therefore redundant, although some understanding of the general views of carers at baseline and follow-up can be surmised from Figure 10.5.

It is striking that, once more, there has been little change between the two assessment episodes. On each occasion the perceived *dependency* of the patient on the carer was the most common experience (scoring a mean rating equivalent to 'often being thought about'). The least of carers' concerns was the *stigmatization* of having a mentally ill relative. The ECI provides some indication of the beneficial elements of caring in the scales *positive personal experiences* and positive aspects of the relationship with the patient (*good relationship*). The importance of this side of caregiving is reflected in the finding that these thoughts come to mind at least 'sometimes'.

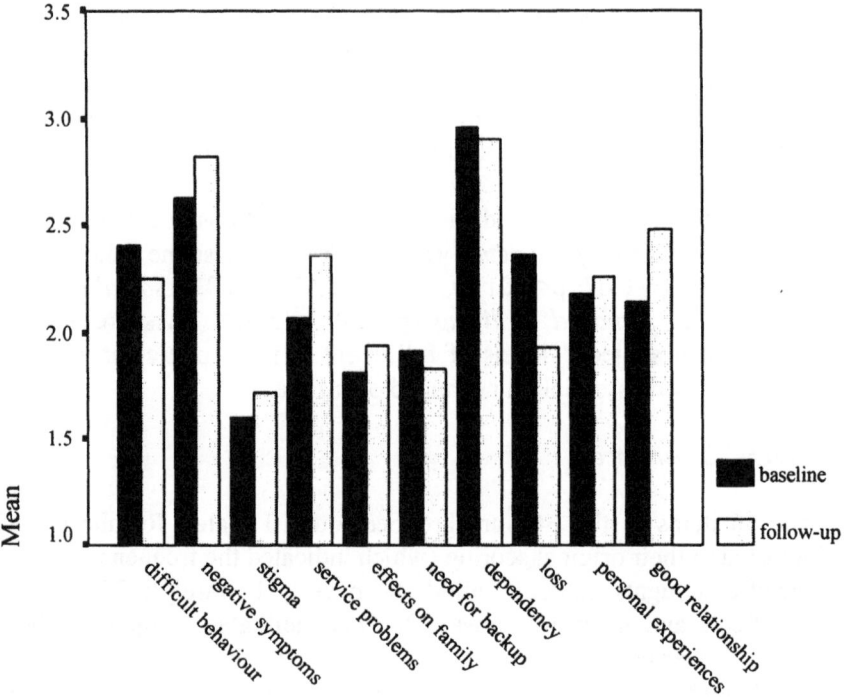

**Figure 10.5  The experience of caregiving: baseline and follow-up**

## Discussion

### Methodological Issues

A number of methodological issues have been raised in this study. The design was, of necessity, a naturalistic and observational examination of the introduction of SEMI registers into a 'real world', rather than experimental, setting. Whilst this has its strengths, the absence of controls has meant causal associations could not be drawn from the study findings. Future research should take steps to remedy this. Other problematical issues which arose in the study, and indeed arise in all studies of people with severe and enduring mental illness, stem from the absence of commonly accepted definitions for basic terminology, such as the expression 'severe and enduring mental illness'. The difficulties which are presented by this have been discussed elsewhere (Barr and Cotterill, 1999a) and one approach to ameliorate the situation is the subject of another chapter in this book (see Huxley *et al.*, chapter 9). The definition of the term 'in contact with mental health services' is similarly open to debate. For example, there is no agreement as to whether this should include only recent face-to-face contacts or those which are less personal and infrequent. Confusion around these terms clearly serves to hinder the progress of research and service development in this area.

*Research Findings*

The findings reported here are based on a preliminary analysis of the data and their import will become more apparent when analysis is completed. Nevertheless, some comment is appropriate in relation to the hypotheses outlined earlier in the chapter.

Firstly, the domains in which the greatest number of subjects expressed need were those of *psychological distress, daytime activities* and *physical health.* These findings were much the same as those reported in similar patient populations by Hansson *et al.*, (1995) and, to a lesser extent, by Slade *et al.*, (1998), in Sweden and South London respectively. In the present study, neither the extent of need, nor the amount of unmet need, was found to have changed significantly between the baseline and follow-up assessments. Clearly, if the establishment of practice-based registers had been instrumental in improving the linkage of registered patients to statutory services, one would expect a reduction in both expressed and unmet need. In the absence of this evidence, we must reject the hypothesis that patients' levels of need for help from statutory services would improve following the introduction of registers.

The second hypothesis held that registers would facilitate improvement in patients' QOL. However, once more, findings failed to support the hypothesis: QOL remained effectively unchanged between baseline and follow-up, and the hypothesis must be rejected.

Because numbers of respondents in the carers' sample were limited, we were unable to apply statistical analysis to results. Although only illustrative, the available evidence suggests that the sense of *stigma* arising from having a relative or close friend with severe and enduring mental illness, was the least of carers' concerns. This was also a finding of Szmukler *et al.*, (1996b), and may suggest this aspect of caregiving is of less significance than many professionals might expect. In relation to findings at both baseline and follow-up, the experiences of carers reflected no sign of appreciable decrease in the burden, nor increase in the positive aspects, of caregiving. This suggests the introduction of registers had little impact on carers and, in all probability, the third hypothesis should be rejected.

If SEMI registers were functioning to their theoretical potential, one might expect a more appropriate use of specialist mental health services by registered patients - the fourth hypothesis. This is because service providers would be seeing the most needy of patients at the follow-up, rather than baseline, assessment. A more appropriate use of services should also be reflected in the reduction of crises in patients' lives, which would be manifest in fewer detentions under the *Mental Health Act* (House of Commons, 1983) and lower in-patient bed usage. At the time of going to press, these data had yet to be fully analysed. However, the study did generate findings concerning the baseline position in relation to contact with specialist mental health services. For example, there was evidence that those patients who were probably the most socially disabled by their mental illness – people with a psychotic diagnosis - were most likely to be in touch with mental health services, a finding also reported by Kendrick *et al.*, (1994); see also Barr, (*in press*). To this extent, findings accord with expectations that mental health services should be targeted on patients with serious mental illness (Audit Commission, 1994; DoH, 1994b; 1995a; 1995b). However, this observation was made at baseline – before the SEMI registers would have had a significant impact on service contact. We are, therefore, unable to conclude that registers are associated with the more appropriate use of mental health services.

Findings do, however, highlight the fact that primary care services are carrying sole responsibility for significant numbers of patients with severe and enduring mental health problems. It is in keeping with government thinking that the primary care sector should be at the heart of care for most patients (NHS Executive, 1996; DoH, 1997). However, there is little evidence that most primary health care teams are prepared to meet this challenge with the SEMI patient group. In fact, the evidence strongly suggests that few teams have developed structured guidelines and policies for the care of SEMI patients (Falloon *et al.*, 1990; Kendrick *et al.*, 1991; 1995; Goldberg and Jackson, 1992; Nazareth *et al.*, 1993b; Lang *et al.*, 1997). The study highlights the need for the introduction of mechanisms to improve the management of SEMI patients in primary care and to assist closer liaison with specialist mental health services (Bindman *et al.*, 1997).

## Conclusion

On the basis of this preliminary analysis of data we must conclude that the study provides no evidence that the introduction of primary care-held SEMI registers has had a significant impact on patient functioning, carer experience, or the co-ordination and use of services. There are, however, a number of alternative explanations for this lack of evidence. For example, the study was based on small numbers of patients in the sub-sample. This hampered adequate statistical analysis and limited the power of statistical tests to discern change over time. Also, a large proportion of potential members of the patient sub-sample either positively elected not to take part in the study or failed to respond to mailed requests to participate. This suggests the sample was not as representative as it may have been. Those people with the more chaotic lifestyles – who may have had the most to gain from inclusion on a SEMI register - may not have been included in the study. The 12 month time span between baseline and follow-up assessments may itself have been insufficient to allow for measurable change to occur in sample subjects, and future research should take this into consideration. Finally, the Register Initiative was introduced into the district under study at a time of great organisational change, including the merger of NHS Trusts and establishment of multi-disciplinary CMHTs. These reforms may have absorbed the attention and capacity of crucial staff members at a time when these energies were needed to fully implement the Registers Initiative. This would account for the extensive evidence from the monitoring phase of the study, that no practice employed registers proactively in the management of care for SEMI patients. It would similarly account for the absence of positive change between baseline and follow-up assessments in the present study.

There are good theoretical grounds for developing primary care-held SEMI registers. We suggest this study has made some in-roads into the practical application of the initiative. Only further research, with larger samples and controlled conditions, will answer the questions raised about the ultimate viability and efficacy of these registers.

## Acknowledgement

We are grateful for the financial support of this project by the NHS Executive North West R&D Directorate.

We would also like to express our gratitude to the service users, carers, practice managers, CPNs, GPs and members the Advisory Group who have helped and supported us throughout this study.

Thanks are also due to Tracy Quillan for her help in producing this book.

# References

Audit Commission (1994), *Finding a Place: A Review of Mental Health Services for Adults,* HMSO, London.

Baker, G.A., Jacoby, A., Smith, D.F., Dewey, M.E., and Chadwick, D.W. (1994), 'Development of a Novel Scale to Assess Life Fulfilment as Part of the Further Refinement of a Quality of Life Model for Epilepsy', *Epilepsia,* vol. 35, no. 3, pp. 591-96.

Barr, W. 'Characteristics of Severely Mentally Ill Patients In and Out of Contact with Community Mental Health Services', *Journal of Advanced Nursing,* in press.

Barr, W. and Cotterill, L. (1999a), 'Defining Severe or Enduring Mental Illness: by Principle or Prescription?', *Journal of Psychiatric and Mental Health Nursing,* vol. 6, pp. 489-91.

Barr, W. and Cotterill, L. (1999b), 'Registering Concern: the Case of Primary Care Held Registers for People with Severe and Enduring Mental Illness', *Health and Social Care in the Community,* vol. 7, no. 6, pp. 427-33.

Bindman, J., Johnson, S., Wright, S., Szmukler, G., Bebbington, P., Kuipers, E. and Thornicroft, G. (1997), 'Integration Between Primary and Secondary Services in the Care of the Severely Mentally Ill: Patients' and General Practitioners' Views', *British Journal of Psychiatry,* vol. 171, pp. 169-74.

Department of Health (1994a), *Introduction of Supervision Registers for Mentally Ill People from 1st April 1994,* (HSG(94)5), Department of Health, London.

Department of Health (1994b), *Working in Partnership: A Collaborative Approach to Care,* Report of the Mental Health Nursing Review Team, HMSO, London.

Department of Health (1995a), *The Health of the Nation: Building Bridges,* HMSO, London.

Department of Health (1995b), *Report of the Clinical Standards Advisory Group on Schizophrenia,* HMSO, London.

Department of Health (1997), *The New NHS: Modern, Dependable,* Cm. 3807, The Stationery Office, London.

Department of Health (1999), *National Service Framework for Mental Health,* Department of Health, London.

Falloon, I.R.H., Shanahan, W., Laporta, M. and Krekorian, H.A.R. (1990), 'Integrated Family, General Practice and Mental Health Care in the Management of Schizophrenia', *Journal of the Royal Society of Medicine,* vol. 83, pp. 225-28.

Goldberg, D. and Jackson, G. (1992), 'Interface Between Primary Care and Specialist Mental Health Care', *British Journal of General Practice*, vol. 42, pp. 267-69.

Hansson, L., Bjorkman, T., and Svensson, B. (1995), 'The Assessment of Need in Psychiatric Patients', *Acta Psychiatrica Scandinavica*, vol. 92, pp. 285-93.

Hassall, C. and Stilwell, LA. (1977), 'Family Doctor Support for Patients on a Psychiatric Case Register', *Journal of the Royal College of General Practitioners*, vol. 27, pp. 605-8.

Hoskins, A and Langshaw, G. (1996), '*Provision of Care to Practice Patients with Severe and Enduring Mental Illness'*, Liverpool Health Authorities, Liverpool.

House of Commons (1983), *The Mental Health Act*, HMSO, London.

Kendrick, T., Sibbald, B., Burns, T. and Freeling, P. (1991), 'Role of General Practitioners in Care of Long Term Mentally Ill Patients', *British Medical Journal*, vol. 302, pp. 508-10.

Kendrick, T., Burns, T., Freeling, P. and Sibbald, B. (1994), 'Provision of Care to General Practice Patients with Disabling Long-Term Mental Illness: A Survey in 16 Practices', *British Journal of General Practice*, vol. 44, pp. 301-5.

Kingdon, D. (1996), 'Supervision Registers: Caring or Controlling?', *British Journal of Hospital Medicine*, vol. 56, no. 9, pp. 470-2.

Lang, F.H., Johnstone, E.C. and Murray, G.D. (1997), 'Service Provision for People with Schizophrenia: 11. Role of the General Practitioner', *British Journal of Psychiatry*, vol. 171, pp. 165-68.

Nazareth, I., King, M., Haines, A., Rangel, L. and Myers, S. (1993a), 'Accuracy of Diagnosis of Psychosis on General Practice Computer System', *British Medical Journal*, vol. 307, no. 3, pp. 2-4.

Nazareth, I.D., King, M.B., Haines, A., See Tai, S. and Hall, G. (1993b), 'Care of Schizophrenia in General Practice', *British Medical Journal*, vol. 307, p. 910.

NHS Executive (1996), *Primary Care: The Future*, Department of Health, London.

Phelan, M., Slade, M., Thornicroft, G., Dunn, G., Holloway, F., Wykes, T., Strathdee, G., Loftus, L., McCrone, P. and Hayward, P. (1995), 'The Camberwell Assessment of Need: the Validity and Reliability of an Instrument to Assess the Needs of People with Severe Mental Illness', *British Journal of Psychiatry*, vol. 167, pp. 589-95.

Powell, R and Slade, M. (1996), 'Defining Severe Mental Illness', in G. Thornicroft and G. Strathdee (eds), *Commissioning Mental Health Services*, HMSO, London, pp. 13-27.

Slade, M., Phelan, M., and Thornicroft, G. (1994), *Camberwell Assessment of Need (CAN) Research Version 3.0 Manual*, PRISM, Institute of Psychiatry, London.

Slade, M., Powell, R. and Strathdee, G. (1997), 'Current Approaches to Identifying the Severely Mentally Ill', *Social Psychiatry and Psychiatric Epidemiology*, vol. 32, pp. 177-84.

Slade, M., Phelan, M., and Thornicroft, G. (1998), 'A Comparison of Needs Assessed by Staff and by an Epidemiologically Representative Sample of Patients with Psychosis', *Psychological Medicine*, vol. 28, pp. 543-50.

Sykes, C., and Smith, J. (1995), *District Audit Review: Mental Health Services,* Wirral Health Authority, St Catherine's Hospital, Tranmere.

Szmukler, G.I., Burgess, P., Herrman, H., Benson, A., Colusa, S., and Bloch, S. (1996a), 'Caring for Relatives with Serious Mental Illness: The Development of the Experience of Caregiving Inventory', *Social Psychiatry and Psychiatric Epidemiology*, vol. 31, pp. 137-48.

Szmukler, G.I., Herrman, H., Colusa, S., Benson, A. and Bloch, S. (1996b), 'A Controlled Trial of a Counselling Intervention for Caregivers of Relatives with Schizophrenia', *Social Psychiatry and Psychiatric Epidemiology*, vol. 31, pp. 149-55.

Tyrer, R, Morgan, L, Van Horn, E, Jayakody, M., Evans, K., Brummell, R., White, T., Baldwin, D., Harrison-Read, P. and Johnson, T. (1995), 'A Randomised Controlled Study of Close Monitoring of Vulnerable Psychiatric Patients', *The Lancet*, vol. 345, pp. 756-59.

# PART 4
# TARGETING INITIATIVES

# 11 Targeting Mental Health Services for Minority Ethnic Groups

GURCH RANDHAWA

## Introduction

This chapter seeks to explore the issues related to providing culturally competent, equitable mental health services for minority ethnic groups in the UK. This has become an increasingly important area of work as research evidence has highlighted the disproportionately higher rates of hospital admissions among African Caribbeans and some of the Asian sub-populations suffering from a mental illness. The chapter consists of a review of relevant literature focusing upon ethnicity and mental health, and draws upon observations from an on-going participatory action-research project, 'Partnerships for Change', which seeks to provide culturally competent mental health services within Bedfordshire. The author of this chapter is a Principal Lecturer in Health Services Research and was involved in the action research project. The chapter begins with a brief background that outlines how addressing the needs of minority ethnic groups has become more visible on the health policy agenda. The rationale for the 'Partnerships for Change' project, and its subsequent development, are then described. This includes a review of the research related to examining the prevalence of mental illness among minority ethnic groups, and a review of initiatives which have sought to provide more culturally competent services. Next, the initial findings from the 'Partnerships for Change' project are presented, and the chapter concludes with a brief discussion of some possible ways forward.

## Background

Over the last twenty years, there has been a shift of focus in health policy that has resulted in a growing interest in the health of minority ethnic populations in the UK. Two quotes summarise this shift. The first quote is one of the key aims of the government's health policy; the second, provides a definition of what is meant by equity in health care.

> To improve the health of the worst off in society and to narrow the health gap (DoH, 1999, p.4).

> Equity in health care would be to ensure equal access and use of available health care for equal need, with equal quality of care for all (Whitehead, 1995, p22).

The 1991 census featured the inclusion of a question seeking to identify ethnic-group. This has aided, to some extent, the examination of health status for different ethnic groups. Government strategy papers such as *Health of the Nation* (DoH, 1992) and the more recent *Saving Lives: Our Healthier Nation* (DoH, 1999), have highlighted the specific health problems faced by minority ethnic groups in the UK, and the need for an urgent course of action to reduce health inequalities. The Department of Health established the NHS Ethnic Health Unit in 1994, which aimed to promote health and healthcare for minority ethnic groups (NHS Confederation, 1998). The Health Education Authority has carried out two health and lifestyle surveys of black and minority ethnic groups, which have sought to highlight information regarding health behaviours and health status (Rudat, 1994). Most recently, the Fourth National Survey, conducted by the Policy Studies Institute (PSI) and Social and Community Planning Research (SCPR), included an extensive section on health among minority ethnic groups (Nazroo, 1997). Throughout this period, the provision of mental health services for minority ethnic groups has become a particularly controversial area of debate. This is in part due to the observation of high rates of schizophrenia among African Caribbean populations in the UK, and high rates of suicide among South Asian women. Further research has been recommended in this area to explore the apparent problems of mental health within minority ethnic groups (Smaje, 1995; Cochrane and Sashidharan, 1996; Nazroo, 1997).

## 'Partnerships for Change' – The Context

The 1991 Census identifies 6% of the UK's population as being from minority ethnic groups. Bedfordshire has one of the most diverse range of communities for any shire county, in which 10% of the population is from minority ethnic groups (see Appendix 1). The county is made up of four distinct areas - Luton, South Bedfordshire, Mid-Bedfordshire, and North Bedfordshire, in which minority ethnic groups comprise 19.8%, 2%, 1.9%, and 10.1% of the population respectively (OPCS, 1992). Furthermore, evidence shows that the majority of minority ethnic groups reside in the most deprived wards within Bedfordshire, and are from lower socio-economic groups – factors which have been shown to adversely affect access to, and uptake of, health services (Smaje, 1995; DoH, 1999). Therefore, an essential first step is for service providers to be appropriately equipped with the local demographic knowledge, resources, and training to ensure that they are able to meet the needs of their local populations. In order to facilitate these developments, the Department of Health and the NHS Executive have funded a two-year participatory action research project in Bedfordshire.

The Partnerships for Change (PfC) project was initiated to complement the recently developed Bedfordshire Minority Ethnic Health Strategy. The main objectives of the PfC are to:

- identify the reasons for under-use and over-use of services by minority groups;
- offer a voice to those in the community who are unheard;
- promote change in the cultural competency of services, in order to move ethnicity from the margin to mainstream of health care delivery;
- increase appropriate access to, and use of, services;
- identify barriers hindering access to, and progression through, care pathways; and,
- identify known effective solutions, at a national and local level, to barriers hindering access to and progression through care pathways.

The PfC project focuses upon three health-related areas: mental health, coronary heart disease (CHD) and diabetes.[1] It is essentially an action research project which is intended to make use of partnerships *between* various agencies to improve the health of minority ethnic groups and, in particular, to move closer to equal access to services for all the communities in Bedfordshire. At an institutional level, its aim is to use

---

[1]In this chapter, discussion will focus on the mental health aspect of the PfC.

partnerships *within* each of the agencies to address minority ethnic health. An essential condition for the success of this project, then, is effective communication between individuals *within* organisations, and *between* individuals across organisations. The main organisations involved are:

- Bedfordshire Health Authority
- Bedfordshire Health Promotion Agency
- Bedfordshire and Luton Community NHS Trust
- Bedford Hospital NHS Trust
- Luton and Dunstable Hospital NHS Trust
- North and South Bedfordshire Community Health Councils
- Luton Social Services
- Bedfordshire Social and Community Care
- Bedford Borough Council
- Luton Borough Council

The partnership organisations involved had a number of key issues to grapple with to ensure a successful starting point for the project. The first of these was to identify the inequalities in access to, and provision of, mental health services that exist in their area; analyse the reasons why they occur; and, establish effective programmes to help tackle them. However, due consideration was given to the fact that in order to 'level-up' the health opportunities for minority ethnic groups in Bedfordshire, even to the average level, would require effort from a range of agencies. Furthermore, it could mean a change in services for other sections of the local population. It was envisaged that this situation would change during the project as the issue of 'ethnicity' moved from the margin to the mainstream of health care delivery.

Therefore, at the outset of the project, a baseline report was commissioned (Paley and Randhawa, 1998) which included an attempt to map the current situation with reference to local and national information in relation to these illnesses which formed the focus of the PfC. The purpose of the mapping exercise was, within the resources available, to:

- identify specific national and local health issues in relation to mental health, coronary heart disease and diabetes;
- review the use of local services in relation to mental health, CHD and diabetes, according to existing ethnic monitoring data;

- review national and local approaches to ethnic monitoring, and identify good practice, where evidence is available; and,
- review the quality of existing local data.

Once these local health inequalities had been identified, the next proposed stage for partnership organisations to consider was to develop a set of targets. In setting targets, organisations would need to decide how these targets would be achieved (including such issues as timescale, resources, and user-involvement), and how the progress towards achieving these targets could be evaluated. For the purposes of this project, involving a number of partnership organisations, it was decided to take a flexible approach to this process. This was so that targets could be expressed in terms of the mechanisms and processes that needed to be in place to effectively tackle local health inequalities, as well as in terms of the desired outcomes.

*Ethnicity and Mental Health: A Review of the Literature*

Inequalities in health care, specifically within mental health services, continue to be reported in the research literature (Dean *et al.*, 1981; McGovern and Cope, 1987; Littlewood and Lispsedge, 1988; Cochrane and Sashidharan, 1996; Nazroo, 1997). A number of research studies over the last 20 years have reported high rates of 'severe mental illness', in particular schizophrenia, among African Caribbeans compared with white people. Diagnosis of schizophrenia has been reported to be at least three times higher among African Caribbeans. In addition to the consequent over-representation of African Caribbeans within mental health services, research has also shown that the use of compulsory orders is much more common amongst African Carribeans, particularly among young African Caribbean men (GPMH, 1992; Koffman *et al.*, 1997, Harrison *et al.*, 1988). However, a number of commentators have cast doubt on these findings as the over-representation of African Caribbean people has been highlighted in research which relies upon hospital admission data, a source of data which has been shown to have a number of flaws (Smaje, 1995; Cochrane and Sashidharan, 1996; Nazroo, 1997). Interestingly, *the National Community Survey on Ethnicity and Mental Health* found:

> Contrary to previous research on rates of treatment, rates of psychosis were not elevated among Caribbean men in this study and were not elevated among young Caribbean men. And, while Caribbean women had twice the

rate of psychosis compared with white women, this difference was not statistically significant and was not as high as expected (Nazroo, 1997, p.87).

For this survey, the data were collected in the home and by members of the same ethnic group, rather than by white health professionals in a hospital setting. Data collection was in two stages: firstly, interviews were conducted with 5,196 people of Caribbean or Asian origin, and 2,867 whites; and secondly, where interviewees showed symptoms of mental illness, a detailed clinical assessment was carried out. The findings from this survey suggest the need for further work in exploring the reasons for over-representation of African Caribbeans in mental health services.

Evidence about the levels of mental illness in Asian people (those originating from the Indian sub-continent) is not consistent. For instance, some research suggests that the admission rate for Indian and Pakistani immigrants is lower than that for the white and African Caribbean populations (Cochrane and Stopes-Roe, 1981; Cochrane and Bal, 1989). Yet, there is other work carried out by Dean *et al.*, (1981) which shows higher admission rates for Indian men than white men. However, there is ambiguity with regards to the prevalence of mental illness. The evidence about the prevalence of schizophrenia is more consistent, although it is (as with African Caribbean people) subject to methodological limitations. Some research shows that schizophrenia is about 1.5 times more prevalent in Asian people than in white people (Dean *et al.*, 1981; Cochrane and Bal, 1989; King *et al.*, 1994). On the whole, however, evidence shows that rates of diagnosis of schizophrenia amongst Asians is lower than their Caribbean counterparts (Nazroo, 1997).

Also, while rates of suicide among most Asians are equal to, or lower than, those of the general population, rates among young Asian women are more than twice that of their white counterparts (Soni Raleigh and Balarajan, 1992; Soni Raleigh, 1996). The main rationalisations put forward to explain these observations have located the high suicide rates as being 'culturally' related to the pressures of the extended family, arranged marriages and patriarchal family structures (Handy *et al.*, 1991; Merril and Owens, 1986; Biswas, 1990; Soni Raleigh and Balarajan, 1992). This explanation clearly places less emphasis on the mental health state of individuals but more on individuals' circumstances. However, other commentators have suggested these pressures are, in fact, not too dissimilar to the reasons for suicide among white families. The difference is that the explanations tend to be anthropologised by professionals for Asians (Soni

Raleigh and Balarajan, 1992; Lipsedge, 1993; Modood *et al.,* 1997; Nazroo, 1997).

While the above literature strongly suggest that ethnicity - and related concepts - are significantly associated with access to mental health services, little progress has been reported in either redressing the balance, or in understanding the reasons for the imbalance. For example, it has been observed that the precise role of ethnicity in access to mental health services is unknown (Nazroo, 1997), and there is every reason to think that this statement can be generalised to other services. Any attempt to draw conclusions is complicated by various considerations concerning the available data. Three broad areas of difficulty can be identified. First, it is difficult to disaggregate the data on ethnicity from other socio-economic and demographic variables (Benzeval *et al.,* 1995; Schulman *et al.,* 1995; Baker *et al.,* 1996; Taylor *et al.,* 1997). Nevertheless, some early attempts to do this claimed to be successful, demonstrating that 'race had substantial independent explanatory power' (Falcone and Broyles, 1994). Second, there are considerable doubts about the viability of 'ethnicity' as a variable in health-related research. On the one hand, the concept is vague, and the trend towards self-description has introduced further ambiguities in classification (Aspinall, 1997). On the other, the use of 'ethnicity', independently of variables related to cultural differences, particularly language, religion and place of origin, is regarded as unhelpful (Hilton, 1996). Third, there are additional reasons for thinking that the value of currently available data sets is limited, largely owing to the inconsistency in the way such data is collected (Schulman *et al.,* 1995; Smaje, 1995; Atri *et al.,* 1996; Cochrane and Sashidharan, 1996; Hilton, 1996; Nazroo, 1997).

*Identifying Good Practice: A Review of the Literature*

Attempts to trace material reporting on, and evaluating, initiatives to improve access are likely to prove disappointing. While such reports do exist (Gaffin, *et al.,* 1996; Basham *et al.,* 1997), the evaluation is often little more than an account of a particular initiative, from which it is difficult to generalise. Similarly, the attempt to identify 'barriers' to equal access frequently generates a lengthy list of possibilities, which do not add substantially to the many reports that have been issued by various health authorities and health care agencies in both the USA and the UK. This is highlighted in a review of research on the effectiveness of health service interventions to reduce variations in health undertaken by the NHS Centre for Reviews and Dissemination (NHS Centre for Reviews and

Dissemination, 1995). The review included 94 studies, 68 were from the USA, 19 from the UK, and 7 from other countries.

The characteristics of ways of delivering initiatives, and features of the content of initiatives that appeared to have potential to contribute to the reduction of variations in health, included using:

- a multi-faceted approach;
- a multi-disciplinary approach;
- face-to face interactions;
- prior needs assessment;
- culturally appropriate interventions;
- peers to deliver interventions;
- appropriate support materials;
- skills development;
- provision of material support and resources;
- prompts; and,
- reminders for use of health services.

As stated earlier, effective communication is essential in providing a culturally competent service. A study of acute psychiatric services at Parkside Health Authority (GPMH, 1992) commented that mental health units do not make as much use of the interpreting service as other hospital departments. This led the researchers to ask: 'How are people whose first language is not English assessed appropriately for compulsory admission?' (*ibid.*, p.85). A study by the Bethlem Royal and Maudsley Hospitals Special Health Authority (Caan, 1993) found that minority ethnic groups made up 27.5% of patients detained under the *Mental Health Act* (House of Commons, 1983), compared with 9.5% of patients who had not been sectioned. Patients who had been sectioned were significantly less likely to understand why they had been admitted. These patients were also significantly less likely to think that the hospital care was beneficial to their health (Caan, 1993). The Parkside study also found that only 51% of people felt that their treatment had been discussed with them and that they had a choice about it. Many of the young black patients said that they felt they had to try not to make trouble for themselves. This included not asking questions about their treatment, diagnosis, and future, and accepting what they were told, even if they did not agree with it (GPMH, 1992). This example highlights the fact that improving communication is not just about providing interpreters, but also about setting people at ease and explaining issues such as diagnosis and treatment carefully. This may have to be done on several occasions, because when people are ill or under stress they are not always able to absorb what is being said to them. For many people, though, an interpreter is essential (McIver, 1994).

Local examples of identifying methods for good practice from Bedfordshire include studies by Allen (1996), Thakoordin (1997) and Chandra and James (1997). Issues identified in these studies include:

- language and interpretation;
- transport;
- the lack of cultural awareness on the part of professionals;
- insufficient public information (with the result that minority communities know little about the services available);
- issues arising from religious practices with which professionals are unfamiliar;
- diet;
- institutional racism;
- socio-economic factors; and,
- traditional forms of medicine used as an alternative to conventional, 'Western' health care.

Though lists of this kind may act as sensitising prompts, suggesting places to start looking in a particular area, there is nothing that can be seen as an authoritative account of the 'causes' of unequal access, or a definitive strategy for reducing it. The implication is, one might suggest, that any authority wishing to make a serious effort to combat the disadvantaging of minority ethnic groups will have to analyse the situation in its own area, and formulate a specific plan, capable of addressing the factors demonstrably at work in that location.

## 'Partnerships for Change' - Baseline Findings and Initiatives

The findings reported here are based on data collected during the mapping exercise mentioned above. The main methods included: a series of interviews with health care professionals, managers, and data services personnel; and, focus groups with members of the community and clinicians. The following barriers to the cultural competency of staff and services were identified:

- lack of awareness of unequal access to services and of services available;
- lack of understanding of local demographics and diversity of communities;
- lack of understanding of culture, religions and languages and how they can impact upon access to health services;
- lack of awareness of quality standards relating to services for minority ethnic communities;
- stereotyping; and,
- Euro-centric assessment tools and advice.

These findings made it a clear priority to develop and deliver in Bedfordshire a training programme that raises issues around ethnicity and health, and encourages the development of culturally competent mental health services. This has been incorporated within the Bedfordshire Mental Health Training Plan by the implementation of multi-cultural awareness training for staff. The programme that has been developed has been designed to provide appropriate countywide training for specific groups of staff. This includes:

- a conference for senior managers from health, social services and voluntary organisations to raise awareness and agree priorities for further action;
- a series of sessions scheduled for qualified staff, including those based within Community Health Teams - these sessions have been designed to raise awareness, and help staff identify issues that need to be considered when planning services and care plans; and,
- a series of sessions for health staff, and one for social services staff, which will focus on the specific training needs of unqualified staff, and raise awareness of issues to consider when meeting the needs of minority ethnic communities.

The training objectives are:

- to review national and local issues on ethnicity and mental health with reference to the national inequalities agenda;
- to recognise the influence of culture and religion on the lives of individuals;

- to raise awareness and understanding about factors which may affect individuals from minority ethnic groups accessing health services;
- to identify issues which need considering when planning services and care plans to meet the needs of minority ethnic communities; and,
- to identify how services can be developed which are based on the perceived needs of communities, and are culturally competent.

The expected outcomes for participants are:

- increased understanding of the value of culturally competent mental health services, particularly in view of the national inequalities agenda;
- increased knowledge about religions and cultures of local communities;
- increased awareness of issues to consider when meeting the needs of minority ethnic communities;
- the ability to provide services which are culturally competent; and,
- short, medium, and long-term action plans, including time scales and a monitoring/evaluation framework, agreed and in place.

As stated earlier, a key finding from the interviews with health professionals was that there was a lack of understanding of how an individual's culture, religion, and language impacted upon their ability to access and utilise health services. Also, there was a perception by health professionals that current diagnostic measures are based on an Euro-centric view of medical care that does not take account of the cultures of minority ethnic groups. Taken together, these findings combine to adversely affect the level of health care provided for minority ethnic groups (Fernando, 1998; Littlewood, 1992). Therefore, the other main initiative of the PfC project is to develop a culturally competent tool for measuring distress in minority ethnic groups.

The underlying principle for developing the assessment tool is that, although the assessment is primarily concerned with the health and physical needs of the individual, this will need to be carried out within the wider socio-economic context of the individual's circumstances. Additionally, there needs to be a shift of emphasis from assessment based on misconceived stereotypes, to an assessment based upon the individual (Fernando, 1998). Specific issues such as overcoming the language barriers during assessment, ensuring that the individual and their family participate in the assessment process, with advocacy support if required, also need to be considered. It is hoped, that by incorporating these factors in the design process, a diagnostic tool will be developed which will provide a holistic assessment of both minority ethnic groups and the indigenous population (Cochrane and Sashidharan, 1996; Fernando, 1998).

## Conclusion

> No real progress towards equality: health of migrants and ethnic minorities on the eve of the year 2000  (Bollini and Siem, 1995, p.819).

This title of an article from the International Organisation for Migration in Geneva (Bollini and Siem, 1995) sets the context for the PfC initiative, which provides an opportunity for Bedfordshire to make a substantial contribution to the making of 'real progress' in targeting mental health services for minority ethnic groups.  Surveying the situation as a whole - so far as that is possible - it is obvious that an adequate programme would need to run continuously, becoming part of the mainstream NHS agenda, and evolve to suit the changing needs of minority ethnic groups. Certainly, it is unrealistic to imagine that the whole range of problems associated with inequality of access will have been resolved in the two-year life of the PfC project. However, as the above findings show, a careful, focused approach is recommendable.  It is better to make progress in a handful of target areas - with the option to evaluate, and the possibility of identifying workable models for successful action - than to attempt too much all at once and achieve little but frustration.

## References

Allen, E.C.J. (1996), *A Study of the Needs of African Caribbean Women*, Unpublished Report, Equal Opportunities Unit, Luton Borough Council, Luton.

Aspinall, P.J. (1997), 'The Conceptual Basis of Ethnic Group Terminology and Classifications', *Social Science and Medicine*, vol. 45, no. 5, pp. 689-98.

Atri, J., Falshaw M., Livingstone, A. and Robson, J. (1996), 'Fair Shares in Health Care?  Ethnic and Socioeconomic Influences on Recording of Preventive Care in Selected Inner London General Practices', *British Medical Journal*, vol. 312, no. 7031, pp. 614-17.

Baker, D.W., Stevens, C.D. and Brook, R.H. (1996), 'Determinants of Emergency Department Use: Are Race and Ethnicity Important?' *Annals of Emergency Medicine*, vol. 28, no. 6, pp. 677-82.

Basham, K.K., Donner, S., Killough, R.M. and Rozas, L.W. (1997), 'Becoming an Anti-Racist Institution', *Smith College Studies in Social Work*, vol. 67, no. 3, pp 564-85.

Benzeval, M., Judge, K. and Smaje, C. (1995), 'Beyond Class, Race, and Ethnicity: Deprivation and Health in Britain', *Health Services Research*, vol. 30, no. 1 Pt 2, pp. 163-77.

Biswas, S. (1990), 'Ethnic Differences in Self-Poisoning: A Comparative Study Between an Asian and White Adolescent Group', *Journal of Adolescence*, vol. 13, pp. 189-93.

Bollini, P. and Siem, H. (1995), 'No Real Progress Towards Equity: Health of Migrants and Ethnic Minorities on the Eve of the Year 2000', *Social Science and Medicine*, vol. 41, no. 6, pp. 819-28.

Caan, W. (1993), *Satisfaction Survey of Special Health Authority Inpatients*, Bethlem Royal and Maudsley Hospitals Special Health Authority, London.

Chandra, J. and James, M. (1997), *Beyond Good Intentions to Action: Community Involvement in Planning and Decision Making*, Unpublished Report by Josam Associates (Bedfordshire).

Cochrane, R. and Bal, S.S. (1989), 'Mental Hospital Admission Rates of Immigrants to England: A Comparison of 1971 and 1981', *Social Psychiatry and Psychiatric Epidemiology*, vol. 24, pp. 2-11.

Cochrane, R. and Sashidharan, S.P. (1996), 'Mental Health and Ethnic Minorities: A Review of the Literature and Implications for Services', in W. Ahmad, T. Sheldon, and O. Stuart (eds), *Ethnicity and Health*, University of York, York.

Cochrane, R. and Stopes-Roe, M. (1981), 'Psychological Symptom Levels in Indian Immigrants to England – A Comparison with Native English', *Psychological Medicine*, vol. 11, pp. 319-27.

Dean, G., Walsh, D., Downing, H., and Shelley, E. (1981), 'First Admissions of Native-Born and Immigrants to Psychiatric Hospitals in South-East England 1976', *British Journal of Psychiatry*, vol. 139, pp. 506-2.

Department of Health (1992), *On the State of the Public Health*, HMSO, London.

Department of Health (1999), *Saving Lives: Our Healthier Nation*, The Stationery Office (Cm 4386), London.

Falcone, D. and Broyles, R. (1994), 'Access to Long-Term Care: Race as a Barrier', *Journal of Health Politics, Policy and Law*, vol. 19, no. 3, pp. 583-95.

Fernando, S. (1998), 'Studies into Issues of 'Race' and Culture in Psychiatry', *Psychological Medicine*, vol. 28, pp. 496-97.

Gaffin, J., Hill, D. and Penso, D. (1996), 'Opening Doors: Improving Access to Hospice and Specialist Palliative Care Services by Members of the Black and Minority Ethnic Communities', *British Journal of Cancer Supplements*, vol. 29, pp. 51-3.

Good Practices in Mental Health (GPMH) (1992), *Consumer Audit of Acute Psychiatric Services for Adults in Parkside Health Authority,* GPMH, London.

Handy, S., Chithiramohan, R.N., Ballard, C.G. and Silveira, W.R. (1991), 'Ethnic Differences in Adolescent Self-Poisoning: A Comparison of Asian and Caucasian Groups', *Journal of Adolescence,* vol. 14, pp. 157-62.

Harrison, G., Owens, D., Holton, A., Neilson, D., and Boot, D. (1988), 'A Prospective Study of Severe Mental Disorder in Afro-Caribbeans', *Psychological Medicine,* vol. 18, pp. 643-57.

Hilton, C. (1996), 'Collecting Ethnic Group Data for Inpatients: Is it Useful?', *British Medical Journal,* vol. 313, pp. 923-25.

House of Commons (1983), *The Mental Health Act,* HMSO, London.

King, M., Coker, E., Leavey, G., Hoare, A. and Johnson-Sabine, E. (1994), 'Incidence of Psychotic Illness in London: Comparison of Ethnic Groups', *British Medical Journal,* vol. 309, pp. 1115-9.

Koffman, J., Fulop, N. J., Pashley, D. and Coleman, K. (1997), 'Ethnicity and Use of Acute Beds: One-Day Survey in North and South Thames', *British Journal of Psychiatry,* vol. 171, pp. 238-41.

Lipsedge, M. (1993), 'Mental Health: Access to Care for Black and Ethnic Minority People', in A. Hopkins and V. Bahl (eds), *Access to Health Care for People from Black and Ethnic Minorities,* Royal College of Physicians, London.

Littlewood, R. (1992), 'Psychiatric Diagnosis and Racial Bias: Empirical and Interpretative Approaches', *Social Science and Medicine,* vol. 34, no.2, pp. 141-49.

Littlewood, R. and Lipsedge, M. (1988), 'Psychiatric Illness Among British Afro-Caribbeans', *British Medical Journal,* vol. 296, pp. 950-51.

McGovern, D. and Cope, R. (1987), 'First Psychiatric Admission Rates of First and Second Generation Afro-Caribbeans', *Social Psychiatry,* vol. 22, pp. 139-49.

McIver, S. (1994), *Obtaining the Views of Black Users of Health Services,* King's Fund Centre, London.

Merrill, J. and Owens, J. (1986), 'Ethnic Differences in Self-Poisoning: A Comparison of Asian and White Groups', *British Journal of Psychiatry,* vol. 148, pp. 708-12.

Modood, T., Berthoud, R., Lakey, J., Nazroo, J., Smith, P., Virdee, S. and Beishon, S. (1997), *Ethnic Minorities in Britain: Diversity and Disadvantage,* Policy Studies Institute, London.

Nazroo, J.Y. (1997), *The Health of Britain's Ethnic Minorities,* Policy Studies Institute, London.

NHS Centre for Reviews and Dissemination (1995), *Review of the Research on the Effectiveness of Health Service Interventions to Reduce Variations in Health,* CRD Report 3: University of York, York.

NHS Confederation (1998), *Composite Directory of NHS Ethnic Health Unit Projects,* NHS Confederation, Birmingham.

OPCS (1992) *1991 Census: Local Base Statistics,* OPCS, Crown Copyright, London.

Paley, J. and Randhawa, G. (1998), *Partnerships for Change: The Starting Point,* Institute for Health Services Research, Report No. 499, University of Luton, Luton.

Rudat, K. (1994), *Black and Minority Ethnic Groups in England: Health and Lifestyles,* Health Education Authority, London.

Schulman, K.A., Rubenstein, L.E., Chelsey, F.D. and Eisenberg, J.M. (1995), 'The Roles of Race and Socioeconomic Factors in Health Services Research', *Health Services Research,* vol. 30:1 Pt 1, pp. 179-95.

Smaje, C. (1995), *Health, Race and Ethnicity: Making Sense of the Evidence,* King's Fund Institute, London.

Soni Raleigh, V. (1996), 'Suicide Patterns and Trends in People of Indian Subcontinent and Caribbean Origin in England and Wales', *Ethnicity and Health,* vol. 1, no. 1, pp. 55-63.

Soni Raleigh, V. and Balarajan, R. (1992), 'Suicide and Self-Burning Among Indians and West Indians in England and Wales', *British Journal of Psychiatry,* vol. 161, pp. 365-68.

Taylor, A.J., Meyer, G. S., Morse, R. W. and Pearson, C. E. (1997), 'Can Characteristics of Health Care Systems Mitigate Ethnic Bias in Access to Cardiovascular Procedures? Experience from a Military Health Services System', *Journal of the American College of Cardiologists,* vol. 30, no. 4, pp. 901-7.

Thakoordin, J. (1997), *Black, Asian and Ethnic Minorities and Mental Health: Conference Proceedings,* Unpublished Report, Luton Committee for Racial Harmony, Luton.

Whitehead, M. (1995), 'Tackling Inequalities: A Review of Policy Initiatives', in M. Benzeval, K. Judge, and M. Whitehead (eds), *Tackling Inequalities in Health: An agenda for Action,* The King's Fund, London, p. 22.

**Appendix 11.1  Ethnic population of Bedfordshire (1991 census)**

| Group | LUTON | | S. BEDS | | MID BEDS | | N. BEDS | | BEDFORDSHIRE | |
|---|---|---|---|---|---|---|---|---|---|---|
| | *Number* | *(%)* | *Number* | *(%)* | *Number* | *(%)* | *Number* | *(%)* | *Number* | *(%)* |
| White | 137,680 | (80.2) | 106,762 | (98.0) | 107,715 | (98.1) | 120,055 | (89.9) | 472,213 | (90.1) |
| Black | 8,412 | (4.9) | 654 | (0.6) | 769 | (0.7) | 3,743 | (2.8) | 13,578 | (2.6) |
| • Caribbean | 6,180 | (3.6) | 327 | (0.3) | 220 | (0.2) | 2,674 | (2.0) | 9,400 | (1.8) |
| • African | 687 | (0.4) | 109 | (0.1) | 220 | (0.2) | 267 | (0.2) | 1,283 | (0.2) |
| • Other | 1,545 | (0.9) | 218 | (0.2) | 328 | (0.3) | 802 | (0.6) | 2,894 | (0.6) |
| Indian | 7,210 | (4.2) | 654 | (0.6) | 439 | (0.4) | 5,749 | (4.3) | 14,052 | (2.7) |
| • Pakistani | 10,644 | (6.2) | 109 | (0.1) | - | | 1,471 | (1.1) | 12,223 | (2.3) |
| • Bangladeshi | 4,635 | (2.7) | - | | - | | 1,203 | (0.9) | 5,838 | (1.1) |
| • Chinese | 687 | (0.4) | 218 | (0.2) | 220 | (0.2) | 267 | (0.2) | 1,392 | (0.3) |
| • Other Asian | 858 | (0.5) | 109 | (0.1) | 220 | (0.2) | 401 | (0.3) | 1,588 | (0.3) |
| • Other | 1,545 | (0.9) | 436 | (0.4) | 439 | (0.4) | 802 | (0.6) | 3,222 | (0.6) |
| **Total Population** | **171,671** | | **108,941** | | **108,901** | | **133,692** | | **524,105** | |

*Source:* OPCS (1991)

# 12 Targeting: The Role of Training

MICK McKEOWN, DAVE MERCER AND SARA FINLAYSON

## Introduction

Concerns have been raised in numerous inquiries and investigations about the effectiveness of services in meeting the challenge of risk management. Examples of catastrophic systems failures can be recited in a distressing litany of preventable homicides or suicides, achieving sensational coverage in the media and, perhaps, disproportionate influence at the level of government. Since the publication in 1994 of the inquiry report into the case of Christopher Clunis (Ritchie *et al.*, 1994), a pivotal event in the history of UK mental health services, over 80 similar inquiries have been undertaken (Howlett, 2000). A number of authors have attempted to collate and review the various themes and recommendations of this welter of scrutiny into service failings (see Sheppard, 1996), aiming to elucidate further the main lessons which ought to be drawn. Howlett (2000) bemoans the fact that most of these inquiries are of national interest, but remain grounded in parochial systems of dissemination. He points out that there is no statutory mechanism for insisting upon widespread recognition and implementation of the key findings. However, the high profile afforded such inquiries has a corollary in a powerful and enduring lay stereotype equating all mental distress with a propensity toward violence and threat. Consequently, practitioners have to attempt the delivery of care sensitive to the expressed needs of service users against a policy backdrop which, at least at the level of rhetoric, is increasingly drawn toward tighter social control.

This chapter will discuss the notion of targeting in the context of training those who provide care for individuals with serious and enduring mental health problems and are deemed to be especially vulnerable or dangerous. The recent prominence of risk as an organising theme in contemporary mental health services will be acknowledged and engaged with critically. It will be argued that an uncritical obsession with risk

219

assessment and management could have some unintended but deleterious consequences for the majority of low risk service users, suggesting a persuasive rationale for the appropriate targeting of systematic initiatives. The authors will draw upon clinical, research and teaching experience in the care of both mentally disordered offenders and mainstream mental health service users. A considerable volume of research over recent decades has demonstrated that people with severe and enduring mental health problems can benefit from psychosocial interventions. These psychological treatments are designed to either reduce environmental stressors or enhance people's abilities to cope, and to ameliorate psychotic symptoms. Training is a key dimension for the support and development of such targeting initiatives in practice. For Gournay and Sandford (1998) "training holds the key to delivering effective services and hence ultimate improvement in quality of life for those with serious mental health problems". However, despite the success of various training initiatives in effectively improving the knowledge and skills of the trainees together with client outcomes for the duration of the course, this has not translated into any significant or enduring impact at the level of service delivery. Despite the wealth of research indicating the value of incorporating psychosocial approaches into routine practice, there has been a failure to achieve this. At best, implementation has been fragmented or, worse, high quality programmes have only been delivered for the duration of specific research projects. Moreover, in-patient services have come in for particularly pointed criticism (Mental Health Act Commission and the Sainsbury Centre 1997). The report of the Clinical Standards Advisory Group (1995) argued that routine ward care was of a generally poor standard and treatment was almost exclusively focused on the delivery of medication. Research into the views of service users has allowed them to express dissatisfaction with in-patient provision, with specific complaints concerning the poverty of the therapeutic environment (Rogers *et al.*, 1993). Similar concerns have been raised in official reviews and inquiries. It is accepted that systematic psychological interventions are rarely provided within hospital settings, and problems with bed occupancy levels, staffing levels and skill-mix, and appropriateness of staff training for the realities of ward work have all been remarked upon.

This chapter focuses on the role of training in interventions with which people with severe enduring mental illness [SEMI] are to be targeted in order to manage risk. The authors have extensive experience in working with this client group in various service contexts. Both Mick McKeown and Dave Mercer now hold academic nursing posts at the universities of Central Lancashire and Liverpool, respectively. Previously they worked with mentally disordered offenders at Ashworth High Security Hospital. Sara Finlayson is a clinical psychologist who has developed her career in individual and family work for clients with severe and enduring problems, and is currently employed by North Mersey Community NHS Trust, Liverpool. Recently, Sara and Mick have worked together with a multi-disciplinary team of staff in this Trust's secure unit, at Rathbone Hospital, to initiate the introduction of psychosocial approaches to care into routine ward practice.

The chapter begins with a brief discussion of the background context of perceived risk and dangerousness attributed to people with SEMI. Next, the utility of psycho-social interventions is described. This will set the scene for a critical examination of training packages designed to support the dissemination and implementation of these psycho-social interventions and their effectiveness to date. The chapter ends with a description of a training initiative conducted by two of the authors (SF and MM) at Rathbone Hospital High Dependency Unit.

## Background

### Risk and Severe Mental Health Problems

Various types of risk exist in modern mental health services, yet the notion of risk is more often than not conceived of in rather singular terms associated with violence and other forms of dangerousness. Though this set of concerns is undoubtedly of major importance for clinicians and services, and captures the public attention, other significant domains of risk are evident. Ryan (1998) researched the perceptions of risk held by various mental health stakeholders, including staff and service users, who reported numerous risks beyond individual dangerousness. Such a standpoint allows a more sophisticated appraisal of risk that also takes account of the vulnerability of service users to a range of threats to their safety and well-being (Stanley *et al.*, 1999).

People with serious mental health problems are proportionally more likely to be the victims, rather than the perpetrators, of acts of violence or aggression, and are at much greater risk than the general population for self-injury, being especially vulnerable to suicide. Steve Morgan (1998) acknowledges the extent to which users of mental health services can become victimised and describes numerous means by which this can occur. He specifically cautions practitioners to recognise self-neglect as a significant hazard facing this client group. Though severe self-neglect has been suggested as sufficient reason for inclusion on a Supervision Register (NHSME, 1994), Morgan (1998) rightly points to the lack of coverage of such risk in the research literature. An adjunct of a tendency to self-neglect can be deteriorating physical health, and this can be complicated by the inability of primary care personnel to effectively engage with or meet the needs of this group of service users. In this context, standardised mortality rates are worthy of serious concern, being more than double overall in comparison with the general population (Allebeck, 1989). Though the figures can be partly accounted for by accidental death or suicide, they also include significantly higher mortality from respiratory disorders and cardiovascular disease (Burns and Kendrick, 1997), both of which are potentially amenable to prevention or remedial treatment.

Other threats to the welfare of service users encompass iatrogenic factors, notably including the untoward, and occasionally fatal, effects of neuroleptic medication. Similarly, negligent or abusive institutional practices, ranging from verbal or physical aggression enacted by staff, to the failure to protect people from the assaults of other patients, can add to the risks of hospital admission. On top of this, once discharged to the community, the ideals embodied in the phrase 'care in the community' can fail to materialise in any meaningful sense. For many service users, their experience of community case management has been unsatisfactory, with an optimum package of care difficult to realise and untoward burdens imposed on informal carers. Beyond this, people with serious mental health problems are typically subject to a range of societal reactions that can culminate in forms of discrimination, stigma, and social exclusion. The long-term consequences can only exacerbate the effects of negative symptoms, such as lack of energy and motivation, compounding people's social problems and leading to further levels of isolation and loneliness.

*Dangerousness*

Contrary to the high profile and often sensationalist media coverage of serious violence and murder committed by the mentally ill, the epidemiological data presents scant evidence to support the simplistic stereotype equating psychosis with dangerousness. The National

Confidential Inquiry (Steering Group of the Confidential Inquiry into Homicides and Suicides by Mentally Ill People, 1996) into homicides and suicides by the mentally ill has consistently reported that people with serious mental health problems are more likely to be at risk of harming themselves, or being the victim of violence, rather than perpetrating a violent offence against others. Furthermore, it would appear that the rate of homicides committed by this group has remained more or less constant since such data has been collected; this despite the advent of care in the community and the retraction of in-patient psychiatric provision. Indeed, Taylor and Gunn (1999) in their recent review of the homicide rates, report an actual decrease in the rate of murders committed by the mentally ill.

Nevertheless, a significant minority of people with a serious mental health problem do commit violent or murderous acts. Here, a broad distinction can be drawn between criminologists and clinicians about the extent to which mental illness is seen to contribute toward violence or wider offending behaviour. The criminological perspective tends to discount mental disorder as playing a significant role in the causation of crime, preferring to rely upon the strong associations provided across large offender populations by various social factors. In contrast to this, psychiatrists have found evidence, in smaller samples, of a relationship between certain defining features of mental illness and violent behaviour. In a review of the literature, Wessely (1997) argues that, though mental disorder alone is a poor predictor of criminality *per se*, hidden amidst the crime figures lurks evidence that men with a schizophrenia diagnosis are twice as likely as those with any other condition to be convicted of violent offences. There also appears to be evidence from self-report studies that the conviction rates significantly underestimate the actual extent of violent behaviour in this group. However, Wessely goes on to conclude that even allowing for these findings, it is structural factors, beyond the scope of psychiatric intervention, which are the most robust predictors of criminal behaviour.

In this sense it is suggested (Bonta *et al.*, 1998) that predictors of offending and recidivism for the mentally disordered need to be informed by more diverse psycho-social perspectives, as opposed to a narrow and reductionist model of pathology. Thus, in common with general offending populations, the criminal careers of those classified as mentally ill are more strongly influenced by contextual, rather than clinical, variables. Foremost of these is a pre-morbid history of offending, compounded by poverty, disorganised family backgrounds, juvenile delinquency, and alcohol or substance misuse (Monaghan, 1993). Further complicating this already complex equation is the notable failure of many researchers to demarcate specific offence categories within the more nebulous boundaries of violent behaviour.

If the predictive validity of clinical variables remains contested, though, contemporary research has yielded some interesting findings in relation to the role of particular psychotic symptoms and the manifestation of violent behaviour. These would include organised delusions (Nestor *et al.*, 1995; Taylor 1993), thought disorder (Gardner *et al.*, 1996), and command hallucinations (Bartels *et al.*, 1991). An early but often cited study by Hafner and Boker (1973) identified a distinction between seriously violent and non-violent schizophrenics with proportionally more of the violent offenders reporting delusions. Similarly, Cheung and colleagues (1997) found persecutory delusions more likely to be associated with violence, and that those people found to be violent were typically angered by their delusions.

The presence of command hallucinations has been linked to hostility (Bartels *et al.*, 1991) and the vocabulary of such voices has been described as qualitatively different from other auditory hallucinations; reported themes include commands linked to aggression, dependency and self-punishment (Rogers *et al.*, 1990). Arguably, most people who experience command hallucinations are able to ignore them but this ability to resist may diminish in the face of prolonged or repetitive exposure (Honig, 1991). Other characteristics of a person's psychotic experiences have also been suggested as important in predicting who might act upon command hallucinations. Juninger (1990) suggests an increased risk exists for those people who recognise the voice as an identifiable person, or who also have delusional ideas linked to their hallucinations.

Regardless of the specific psychotic symptomatology, Link and Steuve (1994) point to the importance of individual interpretations and responses to symptoms in mediating the potential for violence. Such risk factors include the extent to which a person's psychotic experiences precipitate vengeful ideation, a sense of being under threat, or a lack of self control. This reasoning has led to the coining of the phrase 'threat/control overide' (TCO) as an explanatory device for linking psychotic experiences with violent behaviour. In this sense, personal factors which could operate to inhibit a violent response can be over-ridden when various psychotic phenomena are present. Swanson and colleagues (1996; 1997) report further evidence for this association, with a twofold increases in the propensity for violence if a person admitted any of the following TCO experiences:

- believes mind to be under the control of dominating external forces;
- thought insertion;
- persecutory beliefs; or,
- belief that one is being followed by others.

## *Risk Culture in Mental Health Services*

The systems for evaluating and managing risk in mental health services need to be considered within a wider political and social context. Nikolas Rose (1996) has persuasively argued that these mechanisms, dominated by concern with dangerousness, can be located in broader societal trends in the governance of diverse and unrelated forms of risk. In this sense, engagement with risk is a defining feature of contemporary advanced liberal states, flowing directly from governmental attempts to 'conduct the conduct' of others. For Rose, these emerging techniques of government are best understood with recourse to a Foucauldian analysis of knowledge and power, where expertise and professionalism are bound up with specialist claims to 'truth' or ways of knowing.

From this standpoint, psychiatry, or, more interestingly, an entire psy-complex of institutions, knowledge, and para-professionals, is inextricably linked to the surveillance and management of individual or collective behaviour. Hence the history of psychiatry has witnessed an expanding encroachment of subtle forms of governance into various aspects of civil life, with the containment or supervision of the mentally unwell a prominent feature of this. Viewed in this light, the various technologies of risk management are part of a wider panoply of social control. Thus, for Rose (1996), the role of psychiatry has been revised to suit political developments in the organisation of services, such as the shift from institutional to community care, and various cultural shifts, within and without services. The new role is largely administrative rather than curative, and encompasses various tensions arising from competing expectations.

The psy-professionals have to balance pre-emptive work aimed at maximising a normative notion of mental wellness, with the supervision of individuals whose mental health fails to meet the ideal standard, and hence is deemed pathological, amidst a myriad of different institutions and locations which make up modern psychiatric service configurations. Central to these tasks is the administration of risk, particularly within the community. On the one hand practitioners are enrolled in an enterprise of systematic exclusion, whilst, on the other hand, they aspire to ideals of empowerment, consumerism, and choice. Other pressures arise from the operation within health service organisations of a powerful blame culture, insisting that untoward events are avoidable and that individuals ought to be held to account. For Rose (1996), this constellation of factors constitutes a relatively novel development in psychiatry which 'places new political expectations upon the professionals ... and creates new divisions between good and bad patients, clients and users in terms of a calculus of risk'.

## Targeting Training for Front Line Staff

The last two decades in mental health services have witnessed an increasing momentum behind a call to structure services around a range of psychosocial interventions. These are based on an expanding body of research evidence and might be expected to ameliorate much of the diverse risk described above, and especially to assist in the management of dangerousness. The fact that many of the espoused clinical interventions or organisational systems are relatively novel to services, and have yet to be taken up systematically or comprehensively, means that a powerful case has been made, and continues to be made, for targeting training itself.

A critical disposal toward the effectiveness of training in achieving positive changes to routine services, and a wider critique of quality of care, turns attention to the actual process of training and contemplation of sectoral issues in its targeting to date. We will argue that traditional models of training are insufficient alone to significantly affect the uptake and delivery of psychosocial therapies, and that in-patient services in particular have been neglected, meriting a shift in focus for training activity. In place of these older approaches we advocate a specific interactive model of training, that targets whole teams together and is enacted in the actual clinical environment.

*Psychosocial Interventions*

The range of approaches collectively labelled as psychosocial interventions, together with the necessary supporting frameworks of systematic and co-ordinated case management, have become the essential content of progressive multi-disciplinary training courses. The notion of psychosocial approaches shifts the classical orientation of psychological intervention away from a focus on individual, one-one therapies, toward attention to the wider social network of the index service user. In this sense, problems and needs exist interactively between members of close social groups. This suggests a key role for significant others, typically relatives, in either the direct focus of therapy or, at least, in supporting individually targeted psychological interventions. Within the literature, a significant portion of work has concentrated on the quality of relationships in families and the modification of unhelpful interactions which are collectively termed 'high expressed emotion' (EE), typically relying on lengthy engagement in behavioural family therapy (Barrowclough and Tarrier, 1992). More recently, the research focus has turned to the effectiveness of psychological interventions targeted at positive symptoms, specifically hallucinations and delusions (Bentall *et al.*, 1994; Chadwick and Birchwood, 1994; Chadwick and Lowe, 1990; Drury *et al.*, 1996; Garety *et al.*, 1994; Kingdon and Turkington, 1991; Tarrier *et al.*, 1993). In a similar vein, psychological strategies to enhance compliance with neuroleptic medication have been demonstrated to be effective (Kemp *et al.*, 1996).

Stress-vulnerability models of severe mental health problems posit a relationship which has utility in providing a relatively simple basis for explaining the complexity of psychotic disorders, without necessarily offering a causal account (see Zubin and Spring, 1977; Neuchterlain and Dawson, 1984). Within such conceptual frameworks, psychotic symptoms are understood in terms of an interaction between inherent personal vulnerability and environmental stress. Hence, high EE relationships can be seen as an important source of stress, and the psychosocial intervention targets the whole network, if possible, to reduce the impact of stress for all concerned.

Practitioners and researchers involved in the development of psychosocial approaches, usually rely on the stress-vulnerability concept in conjunction with other compatible principles. There is a concerted effort to engage with service users and carers collaboratively, so that they can exercise a degree of control in a therapeutic alliance. This is sustained by a normalising disposition toward psychotic experiences, which are located on a continuum of subjectivity, rather than rigidly demarcated into abnormality and normality. Similarly, the identification of which problems or needs are targeted in therapy is negotiated between the interested parties. The focus on problems and needs can allow practitioners to proceed with interventions when service users reject psychiatric diagnoses. Systematic care planning and evaluation of progress relies upon the deployment of various reliable assessment tools, to elicit relevant dimensions of the client's experience, and detailed formulation of client's problems are agreed upon to underpin the interventions.

## The Thorn Initiative

Following on from the research into the interventions themselves, further studies have attempted to train nurses to apply these treatments in the community, so that they have a better chance of becoming integral to standard practice (Brooker *et al.,* 1994). Building on this early work, attention turned to the question of how to train sufficient numbers of community practitioners, the majority discipline being nursing, to begin to contemplate achieving a substantial infiltration into the workforce. A notable development towards this goal was the establishment of the Thorn Nurse Initiative in 1994, at The University of Manchester and The Institute of Psychiatry. This innovative Diploma course offered psychosocial interventions training to nurses initially, but latterly to multi-disciplinary groups, aimed at training them to provide specialist care for people who have a serious mental illness (Gamble, 1995).

The first three years of the course, funded by the Sir Jules Thorn Charitable Trust, were systematically evaluated demonstrating significant improvements in various dimensions of student learning and key outcomes for service users on their caseload for the duration of the course (Lancashire *et al.,* 1995). From the start, it was hoped that Thorn trained nurses working with the mentally ill would become analogous to Macmillan nurses in cancer care. The course comprised three inter-linked modules covering case management, family work, and psychological management of symptoms, respectively. Broadly speaking, these subject areas have been followed in more recent developments in the provision of psychosocial interventions training. The course places emphasis upon experiential learning, for example, teaching behavioural family therapy skills through intensive role-playing. The participating students are expected to practise their therapy skills with selected clients and families from their routine caseload. Permission is sought to audiotape these sessions, and thorough feedback and clinical supervision is provided in discussion of these cases back in the classroom.

Since the initial period, the number of centres providing such training has been rolled out across the country, with satellite courses in places such as Bath, Nottingham, and the RCN Institute. These centres now typically offer advanced programmes up to Masters level. Specialist issues have started to be addressed, for example, at the Institute of Psychiatry, with a focus on co-morbidity of substance use; and, at York University, with attention to meeting the needs of mentally disordered offenders and their carers. Other leading edge training courses have been developed at the University of Sheffield, where the training activity has been developed in partnerships with service providers in an attempt to address local contingencies. Non-statutory bodies such as the Sainsbury Centre for Mental Health and the National Schizophrenia Fellowship have also been active in developing practitioner training programmes. The Sainsbury Centre, in particular, following the publication of its review of practitioner training, *Pulling Together*, has been influential in addressing issues of core competencies for practitioners in the field, regardless of specific disciplinary affiliation, and the promotion of real service user and carer involvement in training initiatives (Sainsbury Centre, 1997).

In a similar initiative, the North West Region NHS Executive has commissioned a national demonstration project for the delivery of multi-professional training in core competencies for the care of the seriously mentally ill. This programme, managed by the University of Central Lancashire, has developed different models of training whole teams of staff. Of interest is a 'debriefing' approach to training in-patient teams, which is aimed at optimising the integration and uptake of the training into everyday practice. The collaborative initiative between West Midlands Regional Health Authority and Birmingham University has been held up as an exemplary model of good practice in commissioning training (Gournay and Sandford, 1998).

## Problems with Training

One limitation of traditional schemes, such as the original Thorn course, is that the training is invariably delivered away from the environment in which psychosocial interventions are carried out. Despite the heavy emphasis on skills acquisition and supervision of practice, the distance between this activity and the actual workplace has created difficulties. Many of the participants on these courses return to institutions that are inadequately prepared and organised to maximise their investment in the training. Numerous commentators concerned with promoting the widespread uptake of psychosocial interventions have argued for radical changes to the status quo, either with respect to the nature of wider service systems, or of the training programmes themselves, and the necessary collateral activity to support this (Fadden, 1998; Gournay and Sandford, 1998; McKeown *et al.,* 1998).

Arguably, of all the psychosocial interventions, most training effort has gone into preparing nurses to deliver behavioural family therapy. These training initiatives are also notable for exemplifying the problems that arise in establishing the therapeutic interventions in routine practice. Research evaluations have shown that skilled trainers are able to teach family therapy skills to the extent that the graduates of their programmes are able to practise these effectively. Conversely, in those outcome studies not grounded in specific skills training, with the participating practitioners left to rely on their generic skills, the interventions have been unsuccessful. Notwithstanding this evidence that it is clearly workable to train skilled family therapists, Fadden (1998) bemoans the extremely low proportion of caseload taken up with systematic family work for practitioners who have completed specialist training. For Fadden (1998), the under use of available effective treatments is not just wasteful but is indefensible on ethical grounds. In her scrutiny of this state of affairs, she emphasises organisational factors that have impeded comprehensive implementation, and identifies a trilogy of prerequisites to turn this around:

- high quality training;
- ongoing supervision and monitoring of skills in practice; and,
- attention to changing service systems to aid facilitation of progressive developments.

**The Process of Training: A Potential Solution?**

Corrigan and McCracken (1995) present a persuasive case: if the obstacles to delivering change to services are largely organisational, then the quest for solutions must look to the relevant body of knowledge. They urge practitioners concerned with training and development of state of the art interventions to synthesise the lessons from both organisational and clinical psychology. This leads to detailed attention to the process of training, infrastructure and other factors that may support or impede translating the training goals into practice in real service contexts.

For Corrigan and McCracken (1995), the main barriers to these ends comprise bureaucratic constraints, accessibility of effective treatments, and insufficient numbers of well-trained personnel. Examples of bureaucratic constraints include the extent to which staff are unable to engage in therapeutic work because their time is taken up with administrative tasks such as paper work. Other factors include the perennial lack of resources, particularly with respect to staffing. The question of accessibility of available effective treatments goes beyond the blunt issue of lack of training. Arguably, the day-to-day priorities of staff may be inconsistent with those in the minds of the researchers and clinicians responsible for innovative new treatments. Even if this were not the case, accessibility can be hampered by the reporting of research in scientific papers in language impervious to grass-roots staff. Training deficits are just as likely to be found amidst novice practitioners and staff in pre-registration training, as those long established in practice (Corrigan and McCracken 1995, Gournay and Sandford, 1998). Nursing assistants and support workers who may very well provide the bulk of face-to-face interaction with service users are, in any case, unlikely to have received anything other than minimal training.

Corrigan and colleagues, based in Chicago, have devised an innovative model for developing best practice in behavioural approaches to psychiatric rehabilitation, which they have called interactive staff training [IST]. The approach targets the development of whole programmes or systems and tackles organisational barriers and staff characteristics (e.g. burnout, attitudes) directly. The trainers are committed to working with whole teams in their own workplace, and will look to identify and support 'product champions' from the grass-roots to take forward developments in the longer term. Team preparedness, and level of managerial support, are assessed prior to commencing training, and genuine commitment to support the initiative is sought in advance. Crucially, the training is interactive because the guiding philosophy is one that acknowledges mutual expertise, in a way which mirrors the ideal of therapeutic partnership in, for example, family therapy. The 'line-level' staff, those at the grass-roots, are acknowledged as the experts in their own working environment, whereas the trainers bring the possibilities of new knowledge and skills. The interaction occurs when these different forms of expertise are used collaboratively to address the line-level actualities of practice and workplace organisation. In effect, the new knowledge is shaped and adapted to better fit the contingencies of real-life clinical practice, such that any concrete changes to practice have a better chance of surviving in routine practice beyond the cessation of the training. In a sense, this process of effecting change in a step-wise fashion involving learning, feeding-back regarding real life applications, adapting the intervention to suit, and modifying the training input accordingly, is an approach that mirrors some of the features of action research. Hence, this process suggests an appropriate orientation for qualitative analysis of the change process.

One of the key lessons to be drawn from organisational psychology is that the extent to which the personnel charged with implementing any new technology or service development can claim ownership of the scheme is enormously influential in predicting its success or failure. Hence, Corrigan and colleagues' affinity for interactive training is, in one sense, an acknowledgement of this tenet. By synthesising the different forms of expertise brought to the project by both the trainers and grass-roots staff, ownership is facilitated. Moreover, the scenario where a ready-made blueprint for change is imposed on unwilling or incredulous staff, is avoided. The eventual service development which transpires can be seen to grow 'organically' over time such that the actual individual, collective and organisational changes that occur on the route to improved services, may not have been anticipated beforehand. We refer to this process as organic, because the eventual changes to practice arise from within the team itself from an ongoing adaptation of external ideas and models of practice, to render them optimally suited to the specific clinical context in which they will have to work. Essentially, the process can be viewed as evolutionary, proceeding incrementally towards consensual change. The typical alternative is the disruption caused by superimposed change agendas, which, more often than not, are insisted upon without attention to the grass-roots complexities of particular work locations, and are hence doomed to failure borne out of staff resistance or disregard. In this respect, it would seem that policy implementation has much to learn from this model of training.

## Training Initiatives: Organic Training and Development

We have recently delivered and evaluated an organic training approach to implementing psychosocial interventions working with the High Dependency Unit (HDU) team at Rathbone Hospital, Liverpool. This is a secure unit comprising two wards located on a site mainly devoted to general psychiatric rehabilitation. The unit is part of a regional network providing care for people with long term psychotic problems, many of whom would be regarded as treatment resistant, who also have security needs for various reasons. The HDU network provides a level of secure care below that offered by medium-secure services, and was established as a consequence of a review of high-security services, which identified significant numbers of people being detained at a level of security beyond their immediate needs.

The training intervention was led by a nurse lecturer-practitioner [MM] who was a Thorn graduate, and a clinical psychologist experienced in working with psychosis [SF]. The unit had numerous contextual features that rendered it a good place to attempt to implement psychosocial interventions. The admission criteria ensured that the resident client population were exclusively people with severe and enduring mental health problems, and individuals usually stayed on the unit for substantial periods of time, allowing for continuity of therapeutic involvement. Relying on a stress-vulnerability conceptualisation of service users' problems, allowed us to highlight the significant role played by staff within individual client's social networks, and to focus upon environmental stress at ward level, particularly with regard to the multiplicity of interpersonal interactions.

### Ward-Based Training

The training itself was designed for the participation of all members of the team who wished to take part, and participating personnel included an occupational therapist, a social worker, trainee psychologists, junior medical staff, registered mental nurses and, eventually, nursing assistants. A decision was made early on to attempt to train the registered nurses first, and then utilise these staff to roll out the training at a later time to the nursing assistants. Despite there being some good reasons for this, with hindsight the strategy caused some predictable problems. We would now suggest that future training should attempt, wherever possible, to include all members of the team from the start, even if differential learning objectives require some separate training sessions on occasion. By virtue of proportionality within the team, the majority of the participating staff group were the nurses, and the initial evaluation which we report briefly here was undertaken only with them for pragmatic reasons, with the intention of comparing data with other training evaluations which have targeted this group.

All of the participating team members were allocated to small groups of no more than eight. These groups attended weekly sessions of between one and a half to two hours duration for six weeks, in consecutive waves until all the qualified nurses had completed the training. This portion of the training took six months to complete. In this initial programme, the content covered included a broad introduction to the theory and practice of psychosocial interventions, and training in the reliable use of various assessment tools. The final session of the six week block was always aimed at canvassing views on the best means of taking the whole initiative forward, with time allocated indefinitely into the future for ward-based activity to consolidate the training and adapt the new knowledge into practice. Consequently, members of the team met twice weekly with the facilitators, for up to two hours at a time, to address this implementation agenda, focusing initially upon issues which had been identified in the introductory block. The precise membership of these groups would change from session to session, and was largely opportunistic, depending upon which particular staff were on duty.

*Preliminary Assessment of the Initiative*

Although we have yet to conduct a thorough evaluation of this initiative, the early signs are favourable. A range of specific service developments were brought about at ward level. Following our philosophy of organic development, in a process akin to Corrigan and McCracken's (1995) interactive approach, the consolidation sessions tackled the following themes:

- *Establishment of a Ward-Based Model of Psychosocial Care*

The overall focus of the project was to implement psychosocial approaches, largely seen as a community model, into the routine practice of a ward-based care setting. Prior to this initiative the unit philosophy was directed to the delivery of high standard rehabilitation with a challenging client group, but lacked an overarching theoretical basis to encompass the whole team. Historically, the nursing staff had relied upon a number of conceptual nursing models but remained largely dissatisfied with the adequacy of any of these to organise care in the face of such complex needs. In the course of the training and consolidation period the team developed an approach that grounded their care planning decisions and interventions in a model of stress-vulnerability, emphasising the importance of psychosocial stress at ward level.

Hence, particular attention was paid to the diversity of interpersonal relationships on the ward, especially the quality of staff communications with service users. Attempts were made to mimic communication and problem-solving approaches, typically demonstrated in family therapy, in the context of ward-based interactions. A focus upon professional interactions did not preclude developing initiatives to involve and meet the needs of service users' relatives and/or friends during their stay on the unit. Ideally, both professional and informal carers would be involved, in a way that included all of the significant people within an individual's social network for the period of admission.

- *Use of the Systematic Assessments in Routine Practice*

The incorporation of psychosocial approaches has been supported by attention to various techniques of case management. Of crucial importance was the introduction of a systematic approach to assessment and evaluation of outcome. The staff were trained to use a number of reliable and validated tools for the assessment of different aspects of service users' experiences. These included the KGV or *Manchester Scale* for the assessment of mental state (Krawiecka *et al*, 1997), the *Social Functioning Scale* [SFS] (Birchwood *et al*, 1990) and the *Liverpool University Neuroleptic Rating Scale* [LUNSERS] for the assessment of medication side effects (Day *et al*, 1995). Other instruments, more sensitive to the nuances of psychotic symptoms such as hallucinations and delusions, problems around depression and anxiety, or suicide risk, would be selectively employed as necessary. The routine collection of various assessment and evaluation data, and improved team working, has helped to inform care planning, specifically in relation to risk assessment and management.

• *Ward Atmosphere and Quality of Interpersonal Communications*

We believe that this project has impacted upon the quality of staff/service user relationships in a way similar to the improvements in communication and problem-solving skills enacted during the course of family therapy. There is a degree of evidence that staff exhibit a form of expressed emotion in their interpersonal relationships at work which, in a complex way, is analogous to that found in families (Moore *et al.*, 1992). Although there has been no direct measurement of staff and service user interactions, findings have emerged from other sources to support a positive effect. Thus, information from an independent audit across the whole Trust regarding care and responsibility techniques [CandR, effectively, physical restraint] revealed a significantly reduced level of use by staff on the HDU. Essentially, those staff trained in psychosocial interventions appeared more likely to employ alternative means of managing challenging behaviours, with physical restraint representing a last resort.

• *Establishing a Unitary System of Case Notes*

As a consequence of the organic approach, the multi-disciplinary team worked together to devise more effective and useful ways of organising care delivery and recording information. This resulted in a complete overhaul of the existing care plans, medical case notes and written records of the various disciplines involved. What had been a fragmented and relatively disparate collection of professional records was replaced with a unitary, multi-disciplinary information resource, including a detailed care plan. This latter component focuses on a range of issues perceived by the team, and the service user or family member where possible, to be important areas of work during admission to the unit. It is constructed by the clinical team, in the context of specially designated meetings, with as many different perspectives and views as possible incorporated into a consensus.

- *Improving Care Planning*

Following on from the above, a list of problems and needs is drawn up, and between three and five are prioritised at any one time. Relying on the employment of reliable and systematic assessments, these areas for intervention are, wherever possible, clearly defined in behavioural and measurable terms. The problem-focused approach and system of case formulation is helping to address especially complex needs, such as substance use complicating psychosis, the so-called 'dual diagnosis'.

Clinical interventions are written in simple language and progress, that can be graphically presented, is monitored over time. The care plans are reviewed at least monthly to ensure that the formulations are modified as new evidence arises and problems or needs change. The documentary record of these reviews offers a series of written summaries of progress, making medium to long-term estimates of progress easier to undertake retrospectively. This is not always so simple with traditional case notes. The current system now has a logical structure, linking clinical assessment and multi-disciplinary dialogue and planning to a rational set of individualised interventions. This approach renders the written record of care much more of a 'live' document, one compatible with other developments such as the Care Programme Approach [CPA].

- *Developing Multi-Disciplinary Case Formulation*

A novel feature of the care plan, developed by as many people as possible, but always including the primary nurse, is referred to as the 'formulation' because it provides a detailed working hypothesis of problem development and maintenance. In the care planning process, this leads on naturally to informing possible strategies of intervention expressed as measurable goals.

The formulation is vital as it provides a rationale for intervention. It is also significant in attempting to explain problems, and thus separates out the person from the behaviour. The formulations are developed in the context of multi-disciplinary case meetings, involving as many practitioners as possible, as well as the service user if they wish and are comfortable with the process.

• *Increasing the Degree of Participation of Service Users and Families*

We have attempted, wherever possible, to locate our interventions within a collaborative approach to therapeutic alliances with both service users and their families, if they remain in contact. Hence, we endeavour to involve the service user and significant others in all aspects of the care process with which they feel comfortable. This includes, crucially, the process of care planning. If people have difficulties, for whatever reason, with varying degrees of participation, key staff members assume an advocacy role to ensure the various stakeholder perspectives are aired in the context of decision making. This is especially important if the service user or carer view is contrary to that of the team's. An independent advocacy service is also available at ward level. Other developments have involved targeting the special needs of family members of service users detained in secure environments, including the delivery of behavioural family therapy whilst an individual is an in-patient, and then following this up, seamlessly, in the community on discharge.

• *Improving Team-Working and Communication*

These developments have enhanced the ability of the team to track progress or deterioration in individuals, mainly through the greater clarity in the documentary record of care. This ought to improve the quality of liaison with other agencies, and hence the future care of discharged clients. The new notes effectively review the ongoing progress, and summarise this at monthly intervals. Changes to care are recorded together with the rationale for these changes, which should militate against previously ineffective interventions being repeated needlessly in the future (especially important with respect to the prescribing of neuroleptic medications).

The espoused inclusivity of the shift to unitary notes and participative, multi-disciplinary care planning, has improved various aspects of team-working and inter-professional communication. From the outset, the psychosocial approach has recognised the complexity of any individual's problems and needs, attention to which requires numerous inputs, not all necessarily being in agreement as to the nature of the problem or proposed solutions. This necessitates open and ordered discussion of all the relevant material and differing points of view.

Together with other colleagues, we have developed plans to conduct more sophisticated versions of this training approach, accompanied by more rigorous evaluation, employing both qualitative and quantitative methods. We are confident that substantial improvements to in-patient care can be achieved, especially if the contact between the trainers and the team involves a sufficient amount of time. Our current intentions involve attempts to integrate trainers into whole ward teams for up to nine months, where the trainers are established at ward level on a more or less full time basis for the duration of that period. This would enable a whole range of interactive training activity to take place, and vastly improve upon the limited contact time in the study described above.

## Conclusion

It can be argued that, in the main, the progressive introduction of psychosocial interventions into mental health services, and the various training initiatives which have sustained this, have yet to make a significant impact. Furthermore, what efforts have been undertaken have been disproportionately targeted on community staff and service users. In many respects this is understandable and justified: the dominant service philosophy is, rightly, care in the community and virtually all of the relevant evidence-base demonstrating the efficacy of psychosocial approaches has been furnished from community based research studies. However, this state of affairs leaves in-patient care, and the practitioners employed therein, at a distinct disadvantage which is likely to be connected to the observed quality of such services. Given that community care will never equate with the dissolution of all institutional provision (indeed the remaining acute and rehabilitation wards, secure facilities, and voluntary sector accommodation amount to a sizeable provision), it is possible to predict a bleak future scenario unless equivalent attention is given to the training needs of staff working in institutional environments.

It is already possible to identify trends in the health labour market where the posts that are the most difficult to fill are located in hospital wards, and those staff fortunate enough to be in receipt of quality post-registration education are attracted into other jobs, notably in the community, or removed from direct client contact. The result is an increasing ghettoisation of in-patient services, with the quality of care threatened by the 'double whammy' of inadequate training and workload pressures, not least those arising from a changing admissions profile with the emphasis on those people with the most serious and challenging needs.

It is also not uncommon for these circumstances to co-exist with a less than ideal physical environment, either poorly designed for the task in hand, or simply in need of refurbishment.

High quality training has the potential to address these problems, and move us toward the lauded ideal of seamless services and national parity of standards. We strongly argue that the opportunity to effect progressive change will be missed unless the legitimate calls for an increased volume of training do not also pay attention to the process of the training itself and the settings in which this needs to happen.

# References

Allebeck, P. (1989), 'Schizophrenia: a Life Shortening Disease', *Schizophrenia Bulletin*, vol. 15, pp. 81-9.

Barrowclough, C. and Tarrier, N. (1992), 'Interventions with Families', in M. Birchwood and N. Tarrier (eds), *Innovations in the Psychological Management of Schizophrenia*, Wiley, London.

Bartels, J., Drake, R., Wallach, M. and Freeman, D. (1991), 'Characteristic Hostility in Schizophrenic Outpatients', *Schizophrenia Bulletin*, vol. 17, pp. 763-71.

Bentall, R., Haddock, G. and Slade, P. (1994), 'Cognitive Behavior Therapy for Persistent Auditory Hallucinations: From Theory to Therapy', *Behavior Therapy*, vol. 25, pp. 51-66.

Birchwood, M., Smith, J., Cochrane, R., Wetton, S. and Copestake, S. (1990), 'The Social Functioning Scale: The Development and Validation of a Scale of Social Adjustment for Use in Family Intervention Programmes With Schizophrenic Patients', *British Journal of Psychiatry*, vol. 157, pp. 853-9.

Bonta, J., Law, M. and Hanson, K. (1998), 'The Prediction of Criminal and Violent Recidivism Among Mentally Disordered Offenders', *Psychological Bulletin*, vol. 123, pp. 123-4.

Brooker, C., Falloon, I., Butterworth, A., Goldberg, D., Graham-Hole, V. and Hillier, V. (1994), 'The Outcome of Training Community Psychiatric Nurses to Deliver Psychosocial Intervention', *British Journal of Psychiatry*, vol. 165, pp. 222-30.

Burns, T. and Kendrick, T. (1997), 'The Primary Care of Patients with Schizophrenia: A Search for Good Practice', *British Journal of General Practice*, vol. 47, pp. 515-20.

Chadwick, P. and Birchwood, M. (1994), 'The Omnipotence of Voices: A Cognitive Approach to Auditory Hallucinations', *British Journal of Psychiatry*, vol. 164, pp. 190-201.

Chadwick, P. and Lowe, C. (1990), 'The Measurement and Modification of Delusional Beliefs', *Journal of Consulting and Clinical Psychology*, vol. 58, pp. 225-32.

Cheung, P., Schweitzer, I., Crowley, K. and Tuckwell, V. (1997), 'Violence and Schizophrenia: Role of Hallucinations and Delusions', *Schizophrenia Research*, vol. 26, pp. 181-90.

Clinical Standards Advisory Group Committee on Schizophrenia (1995), *Clinical Standards Advisory Group: Schizophrenia. Volume 1*. Report of a CSAG Committee on Schizophrenia, HMSO, London.

Corrigan, P. and McCracken, S. (1995), 'Psychiatric Rehabilitation and Staff Development: Educational and Organisational Models', *Clinical Psychology Review*, vol. 15, pp. 699-719.

Day, J., Wood, G., Dewey, M. and Bentall, R. (1995), 'A Self Rating Scale for Measuring Neuroleptic Side Effects: Validation in a Group of Schizophrenic Patients', *British Journal of Psychiatry*, vol. 166, pp. 650-3.

Drury, V., Birchwood, M., Cochrane, R. and MacMillan, F. (1996), 'Cognitive-Behaviour Therapy for Acute Psychosis', *British Journal of Psychiatry*, vol. 169, pp. 593-607.

Fadden, G. (1998), 'Family Intervention', in C. Brooker and J. Repper (eds), *Serious Mental Health Problems in the Community*, Balliere Tindall, London.

Gamble, C. (1995), 'The Thorn Nurse Training Initiative', *Nursing Standard*, vol. 9, no. 15, pp. 31-4.

Gardner, W., Lidz, C., Mulvey, E. and Shaw, E. (1996), 'Clinical Versus Actuarial Predictions of Violence in Patients with Mental Illness', *Journal of Consulting and Clinical Psychology*, vol. 64, pp. 602-9.

Garety, P., Kuipers, L., Fowler, D., Chamberlain, F. and Dunn, G. (1994), 'Cognitive Behavioural Therapy for Drug-Resistant Psychosis', *British Journal of Medical Psychology*, vol. 67, pp. 259-71.

Gournay, K. and Sandford, T (1998), 'Training for the Workforce', in C. Brooker and J. Repper (eds), *Serious Mental Health Problems in the Community*, Bailliere Tindall, London.

Hafner, H. and Boker, W. (1973), *Crimes of Violence by Mentally Abnormal Offenders*, (Trans. H. Marshall, 1982), Cambridge University Press, Cambridge.

Honig, A. (1991), 'Psychotherapy with Command Hallucinations in Chronic Schizophrenia: The Use of Action Techniques Within a Surrogate Family Setting', *Journal of Group Psychotherapy, Psychodrama and Sociometry*, vol. 44, no. 1, pp. 3-18.

Howlett, M. (2000), 'Victims and Survivors', in D. Mercer, T. Mason, M. McKeown and G. McCann (eds), *Forensic Mental Health Care: A Case Study Approach*, Churchill Livingstone, Edinburgh.

Juninger, J. (1990), 'Predicting Compliance with Command Hallucinations', *American Journal of Psychiatry*, vol. 147, pp. 245-7.

Kemp, R., Hayward, P., Applewhaite, G., Everitt, B. and David, A. (1996), 'Compliance Therapy in Psychotic Patients: A Randomised Controlled Trial', *British Medical Journal*, vol. 312, pp. 345-9.

Kingdon, D. and Turkington, D. (1991), 'Preliminary Report: The Use of Cognitive Behaviour Therapy and a Normalizing Rationale in Schizophrenia', *Journal of Nervous and Mental Disease*, vol. 179, pp. 207-11.

Krawiecka, M., Goldberg, D. and Vaughan, M. (1997), 'A Standardised Psychiatric Assessment Scale for Rating Chronic Psychiatric Patients', *Acta Psychiatrica Scandinavica*, vol. 55, pp. 299-308.

Lancashire, S., Haddock, G., Tarrier, N., Baguley, I., Butterworth, A. and Brooker, C. (1995), 'The Impact of Training Community Psychiatric Nurses to use Psychosocial Interventions with People who have Serious Mental Health Problems: The Thorn Nurse Training Project', *The International Journal of Psychiatric Nursing Research*, vol. 2, no. 1, pp. 124-33.

Link, B. and Steuve, A. (1994), 'Psychotic Symptoms and the Violent/Illegal Behaviour of Mental Patients Compared to Community Controls', in J. Monahan and H. Steadman (eds), *Violence and Mental Disorder: Developments in Risk Assessment*, University of Chicago Press, Chicago, pp. 101-36.

McKeown, M., McCann, G. and Bentall, R. (1998), 'Time for Action: A New System of Training Mental Health Practitioners', *Mental Health Care*, vol. 1, no. 5, pp. 158.

Mental Health Act Commission and the Sainsbury Centre (1997), *The National Visit*, The Sainsbury Centre for Mental Health, London.

Monahan, J. (1993), 'Mental Disorder and Violence: Another Look', in S. Hodgins (ed), *Mental Disorder and Crime*, Sage, Newbury Park CA, pp. 287-302.

Moore, E., Ball, R. and Kuipers, L. (1992), 'Expressed Emotion in Staff Working with the Long-Term Adult Mentally Ill', *British Journal of Psychiatry*, vol. 161, pp. 802-8.

Morgan, S. (1998), 'The Assessment and Management of Risk', in C. Brooker and J. Repper (eds), *Serious Mental Health Problems in the Community*, Bailliere Tindall, London.

National Health Service Management Executive (1994), *Introduction of Supervision Registers for Mentally Ill People*, HSG(94)5, Department of Health, London.

Nestor, P., Haycock, J., Doiron, S., Kelly, J. and Kelly, D. (1995), 'Lethal Violence and Psychosis', *Bulletin of American Academic Psychiatry and Law*, vol. 23, pp. 331-41.

Neuchterlain, K. and Dawson, M. (1984), 'A Heuristic Vulnerability-Stress Model of Schizophrenic Episodes', *Schizophrenia Bulletin*, vol. 10, pp. 300-12.

Ritchie, J., Dick, D. and Lingham, R. (1994), *Report of the Inquiry into the Care and Treatment of Christopher Clunis*, HMSO, London.

Rogers, R., Gillis, J., Turner, E. and Frise-Smith, T. (1990), 'The Clinical Presentation of Command Hallucinations in a Forensic Population', *American Journal of Psychiatry*, vol. 147, pp. 1304-7.

Rogers, A., Pilgrim, D. and Lacey, R. (1993), *Experiencing Psychiatry: Users' Views of Services*, Macmillan in association with MIND Publications, London.

Rose, N. (1996), 'Psychiatry as a Political Science: Advanced Liberalism and the Administration of Risk', *History of the Human Sciences*, vol. 9, no. 2, pp. 1-23.

Ryan, T. (1998), 'Perceived Risk Associated with Mental Illness: Beyond Homicide and Suicide', *Social Science and Medicine*, vol. 46, no. 2, pp. 287-97.

Sainsbury Centre (1997), *Pulling Together: The Future Roles and Training of Mental Health Staff*, Sainsbury Centre, London.

Sheppard, D. (1996), *Learning the Lessons: Mental Health Inquiry Reports Published in England and Wales Between 1969 and 1996 and their Recommendations for Improving Practice*, (2nd edition), The Zito Trust, London.

Stanley, N., Manthorpe, J. and Penhale,B. (eds) (1999), *Institutional Abuse: Perspectives Across the Life Course*, Routledge, London.

Steering Group of the Confidential Inquiry into Homicides and Suicides by Mentally Ill People (1996), *Report of the Confidential Inquiry into Homicides and Suicides by Mentally Ill People*, Royal College of Psychiatrists, London.

Swanson, J., Borum, R., Swartz, M. and Monahan, J. (1996), 'Psychotic Symptoms and Disorders and the Risk of Violent Behaviour in the Community', *Criminal Behaviour and Mental Health*, vol. 6, pp. 309-29.

Swanson, J., Estroff, S., Swartz, M., Borum, R., Lachiotte, W., Zimmer, C. and Wagner, R. (1997), 'Violence and Severe Mental Disorder in Clinical and Community Populations', *Psychiatry*, vol. 60, pp. 1-22.

Tarrier, N., Beckett, R., Harwood, S., Baker, A., Yusupoff, L. and Ugarteburu, I. (1993), 'A Trial of Two Cognitive-Behavioural Methods of Treating Drug-Resistant Residual Psychotic Symptoms in Schizophrenic Patients I: Outcome', *British Journal of Psychiatry*, vol. 162, pp. 524-32.

Taylor, P. (1993), 'Schizophrenia and Crime: Distinctive Patterns in Association', in S. Hodgins (ed), *Mental Disorder and Crime*, Sage, Newbury Park CA, pp. 63-85.

Taylor, P. and Gunn, J. (1999), 'Homicides by People with Mental Illness: Myth and Reality', *British Journal of Psychiatry*, vol. 174, pp. 9-14.

Wessely, S. (1997), 'The Epidemiology of Crime, Violence and Schizophrenia', *British Journal of Psychiatry*, vol. 170, (supplement 32), pp. 8-11.

Zubin, J. and Spring, B. (1977), 'Vulnerability: A New View of Schizophrenia', *Journal of Abnormal Psychology*, vol. 86, pp. 260-6.

# 13 The Management of Mental Health in Primary and Secondary Care

MARK AGIUS AND JOHN BUTLER

## Introduction

The effective management of mental illness in primary care relies, in large part, on the knowledge and skills of the primary health care team, and their links with secondary care mental health professionals. According to national mental health policy, most mental health problems can, and should, be managed within primary care, whilst people with serious mental illness may require input from specialist secondary services. This chapter describes a series of educational initiatives for primary care doctors and nurses in Bedfordshire aimed at improving primary care psychiatry, and joint-working at the interface between community mental health teams and primary care teams. In 1999, the Department of Health awarded this work NHS Beacon status. The educational initiatives were carried out by a team consisting of a doctor (MA), with a background in general practice who had opted to become a staff psychiatrist in the local community Trust, and a lead community mental health nurse (JB). The chapter is essentially a description of how and why the project evolved and, hopefully, it will give guidance on how to apply the same principles in other parts of the country.

## The Need for Primary Health Care Team Education

At least 95% of mental health issues presenting in general practice are dealt with completely within general practice. The other 5% are referred to secondary care, but most of these will, in the long term, be managed by workers from both the primary care team (PCT) and the community mental health team (CMHT) working in co-operation. This represents a major workload for PCTs, which in a number of ways are disadvantaged in dealing with mental health issues (Goldberg and Gournay, 1997). Firstly, most primary care workers have relatively little first hand knowledge of psychiatry. Only about one third of GPs are believed to have done a psychiatric placement as part of their GP training, and such placements are often not an ideal way of learning about the psychiatric problems they will encounter in general practice. Most primary care nurses are 'general trained' and will have received very little teaching on mental health issues (Onyett *et al.*, 1996). Secondly, although an "evidence base" exists to inform appropriate treatment decisions in mental health, thus far little has been done to use the knowledge in implementing good practice. Furthermore, GPs are constantly bombarded by conflicting claims about drug treatments from pharmaceutical representatives. Our own observations in South Bedfordshire reveal that while GPs are anxious to preserve their counselling services, they are also often unsure about the potential benefits of new psychological techniques such as cognitive behaviour therapy. Finally, it has been suggested that often primary care doctors and nurses, may by likely to under-diagnose depression and other mental illness (Paykell and Priest, 1992; Kessler *et al.*, 1999).

In 1997, to address these issues, we embarked on the planning phase of an educational initiative in South Bedfordshire. At that time, the situation in South Bedfordshire mirrored many of the problems identified above. Most general practitioners in the area relied extremely heavily on the local CMHTs for assistance in meeting the mental health needs of their patients. The consequence was that CMHTs received a very large proportion of requests for counselling services that did not fall within their remit. The exception to this was a few fundholding practices that had invested heavily in counselling services. In general, there was very little evidence of interchange of information between primary care and secondary mental health services, except in the form of letters between the CMHTs and the PCTs. There was also little evidence that there was an awareness of modern mental health care methods among PCTs. For example, it was clear that GPs were often using tricyclic antidepressants at inappropriately low dosage; were still dubious about using selective serotonin reuptake inhibitors (SSRI); did not understand the need for the use of atypical antipsychotics; and, had no knowledge of, nor access to, cognitive behaviour therapy. The newer anti-depressants and anti-psychotics offer important advantages in terms of greater efficiency and fewer side effects. On the other hand, CMHTs had been told to concentrate on treating people with serious mental illness (SMI), but struggled with a large number of "inappropriate" referrals. With one or two notable exceptions, community mental health nurses (CMHN) had received no training in cognitive therapy, and were mostly seen as "depot injection nurses". Also, Family Therapy was unavailable to families with seriously mentally ill patients.


## Developing an Educational Initiative

In developing an educational initiative in South Bedfordshire, we attempted to educate the various components of the mental health system, and then to organisationally rationalise the system. This was intended to produce a more effective system that is totally integrated and capable of meeting all the mental health needs of the population in a seamless fashion. In this system, less serious mental health problems will be dealt with effectively at primary care level; while serious mental illness will draw on the resources of both primary and secondary care, brought together in a coherent way.

It was decided that an educational initiative aimed at primary care doctors and nurses would be beneficial in:

- enhancing the ability of GPs and their practice nurses in diagnosing common mental health conditions such as depression, dementia or early psychosis;
- enabling GPs and primary care nurses to be more effective in managing mental health conditions; and,
- creating an atmosphere wherein co-operation between PCTs and CMHTs is enhanced.

In order to develop a strategy for applying our educational initiative, it was important to develop a theoretical model of what an evidence-based seamless service would look like. Essentially, communication across the primary/secondary care interface was the key to the model, and it was clear that one person would have to take on the role of being the 'communication channel' between the two teams. We visited several sites where such teams were being developed, and considered the evidence regarding the 'consultation-liaison' model discussed by Gask *et al.* (1997). It was clear that the person best placed to provide the liaison link between the CMHT and the PCT was the CMHN, who was a member of both teams. In this position, the CMHN could deal with people with SMI in the practice as a case manager. The CMHN could also act as a link between the psychiatrist and the GP, as well as giving advice directly to the GP. The CMHN would have access to the GP's notes and computer system; could ensure that the practice had a CPA register; and, ensure that all CPA2 patients had care plans which were known to the GP. In addition, the CMHN could give clinical supervision to primary care nurses who might be dealing with people with less serious mental health problems in the practice. In order to do this, the CMHNs would need to be qualified as case managers, and trained in:

- risk assessment;
- cognitive therapy for psychosis (which may help modify the patient's perception of delusions and hallucinations);
- family therapy in SMI (which has been shown to minimise relapse); and
- compliance therapy (which is a form of motivational interviewing to encourage patients to take their medication regularly, and so helps prevent a relapse of the illness).

It is well established that primary care nurses have a role in identifying and helping manage anxiety and depression, identifying dementia and identifying postnatal depression, as well as potentially identifying patients with psychotic symptoms (Mann *et al.,* 1998). Thus, practice nurses, district nurses and health visitors all have a potential role in mental health practice. To fulfil this role, they need training, support and clinical supervision, all of which the CMHN is well placed to provide.

In Figure 13.1, we have developed a theoretical model of a seamless mental health service, which helps to identify the roles of each member of the PCT and the CMHT, and highlights their training requirements. It is essential that all the members of the PCT take on a role in dealing with mental health problems, or the team will find it impossible to deal with this major burden in day-to-day practice. Practice councillors will also play a useful role, so long as their interventions are seen to be evidence-based and effective.

The next stage for the education team was to undergo approved training in educating PCTs. The authors were both fortunate in receiving sponsorship to join the program for training Mental Health Facilitators, run jointly by the Royal College of General Practitioners and the Institute of Psychiatry. The course organisers are Dr Andre Tylee (see Tylee, 1999), Senior Fellow in Mental Health at the RCGP, and Mrs Elizabeth Armstrong, Head of the National Centre for Educating Practice Nurses on Depression. The course is run as a number of modules over a period of one year. Between modules, trainee facilitators begin to engage with practices, and are given supervision of their work in the modules. It is intended that the trainees work in doctor/ nurse pairs so that, in visiting a practice, they are able to engage with the whole PCT. In turn, it is hoped that the PCT will work together to develop better systems within their practice to deal with mental health problems.

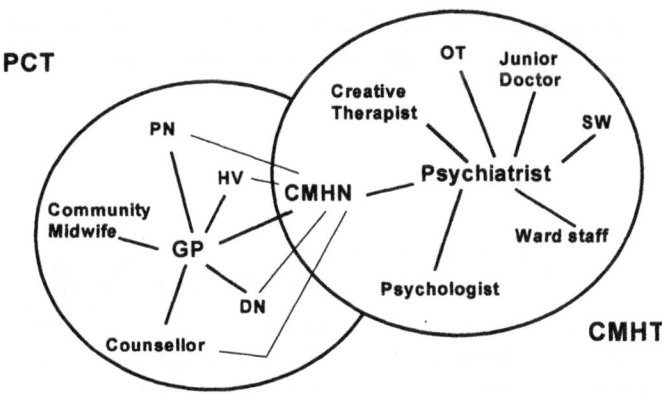

**Figure 13.1    The liaison model**

In visiting practices, we found that it was often very difficult to persuade a PCT to admit to having any particular problems. However, when they did, it was then possible to enable the team to put together a plan in order to improve practice in the identified area. The facilitation team would deliver an educational intervention based on the package it had devised, and monitor progress.

Thus, in a range of practices, different educational interventions were delivered. These included interventions aimed at:

- the identification and management of postnatal depression;
- how to deal with aggressive patients;
- training the practice nurses to identify patients who presented with depression; and,
- showing practice nurses how to deal with problems related to anxiety.

We identified participating PCTs by writing to all general practices in the Luton and Dunstable areas to offer our services. In the first year, we visited six practices. Others were included later on. In each practice we visited, we wrote a report of our conversation with the team for our records. This served as our assessment of the practice, and contained bullet points identifying the areas on which we agreed to work with the practice. This report was shared with the practice and used as a basis for our future work with the practice team. Figure 13.2 shows the work of the mental health facilitators across the primary care/ secondary mental health services interface.

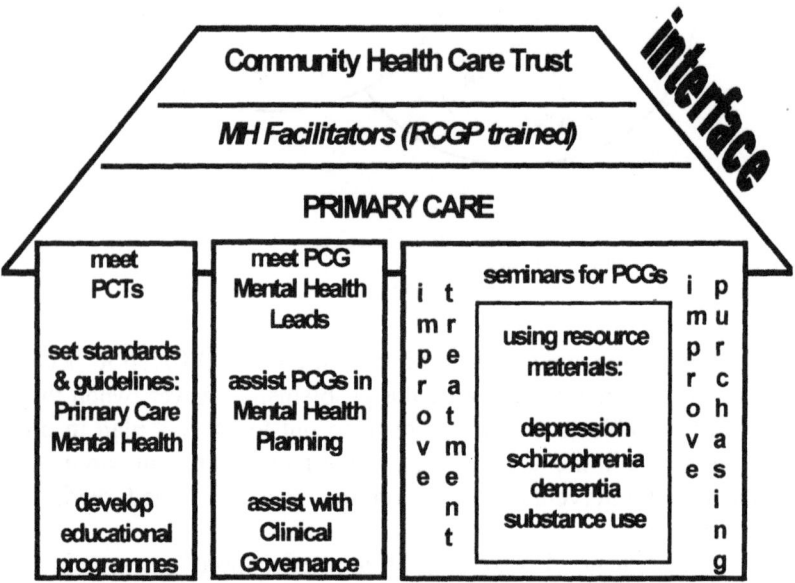

**Figure 13.2    Clinical governance:  across the interface**

As our practice visits grew in number, it became apparent that certain issues were arising time and again. Therefore, we began to develop packages of guidelines on basic mental health problems that we could use repeatedly. Each pack contained a set of guidelines, information from scientific papers on which they were based, and copies of the overheads which we might use in a presentation on the subject. All our packages contain information on diagnosis and information on treatment, including both pharmaceutical and cognitive behavioural treatment.

The packages we have produced include:

- The Identification and Management of Depression in Primary Care;
- Joint working between the CMHT and Primary Care in Schizophrenia;
- The Identification and Management of Dementia in Primary Care;
- The Identification and Management of Postnatal Depression in Primary Care;
- Alcohol Problems in Primary Care;
- Anxiety Management in Primary Care; and,
- Information on the Care Programme Approach (CPA).

We realised that it would be a good idea to organise workshops for PCTs (both GPs and nurses) in which we could address several practices together. We used the packages described above as the basis of these workshops, and each participant received a copy of the package. We began with a series of workshops on depression, and then we added a series of workshops on schizophrenia. More recently, we have started two more series of workshops, one on the management of dementia, and one on the management of alcohol problems in primary care. By the end of 1998, we had presented workshops involving 25 practices in two primary care group (PCG) areas, including 26 GPs and 20 practice nurses. The content of our workshops is shown below.

A typical Depression Workshop will deal with:

- the recognition of depression;
- assessment of suicide risk;
- introduction to management techniques, including medication, cognitive-behavioural and social interventions;
- video exercises including pre-recorded vignettes;
- co-ordination of primary care interventions and CMHT interventions; and,
- general discussion.

A typical Schizophrenia Workshop will include:

- diagnosis and natural course of schizophrenia;

- principles of the Care Program Approach;
- the role of the consultant and the CMHT;
- the role of the GP and the PCT;
- developing joint protocols;
- introduction to management with medication and psychosocial interventions; and,
- summary and discussion.

A typical Dementia Workshop includes:

- identification of dementia;
- the different forms of dementia;
- appropriate investigations;
- screening and the over 75 check;
- medication for symptom control;
- the new drugs; and,
- the roles of nursing staff, OT and social services.

A typical Alcohol Workshop includes:

- the problems caused by alcohol;
- screening for alcohol consumption;
- the issue of dual diagnosis;
- motivational interviewing;
- the role of drugs in management; and,
- other cognitive-behavioural interventions in dual diagnosis.

At the request of a number of practices, we undertook to run an educational workshop programme for practice nurses in the Luton PCG area. In this series of workshops, lasting 5 sessions, we were able to train practice nurses to identify depression in their primary care work, and then teach them some basic cognitive-behavioural techniques such as problem solving for managing depression. Then, we moved on to the identification and management of anxiety-based problems. We hope to repeat the success of this course in other groups of practices.

In order to gauge the level of support by primary care nurses for training in mental health topics, our team, in conjunction with the Audit Department of the Trust and the Bedfordshire Audit and Education Group (BAEG), distributed a questionnaire to all practice nurses, district nurses and health visitors in South Bedfordshire.

The results of this activity showed that:

- health visitors wished for more training on post-natal depression;
- district nurses wished to know about dementia;
- all three groups wished for training on depression and substance abuse;
- all three groups wanted advice about when to refer patients; and,
- most primary nurses did not know about the CPA process and did not know the liaison CMHN attached to their practice.

Funding has been sought from the Bedfordshire Consortium to provide training on all these aspects of mental health care. In South Bedfordshire, our team has been able to distribute registers of CPA2 patients to all practices via their liaison CMHN every three months, and so to involve practices in the CPA process. In order to support our programme, we are developing computerised audit packages for use in both primary care and the CMHTs, to audit the management of depression in primary care and of schizophrenia and depression in the CMHTs. This is a local development of a major audit of schizophrenia in the CMHTs undertaken on our behalf by a commercial organisation.

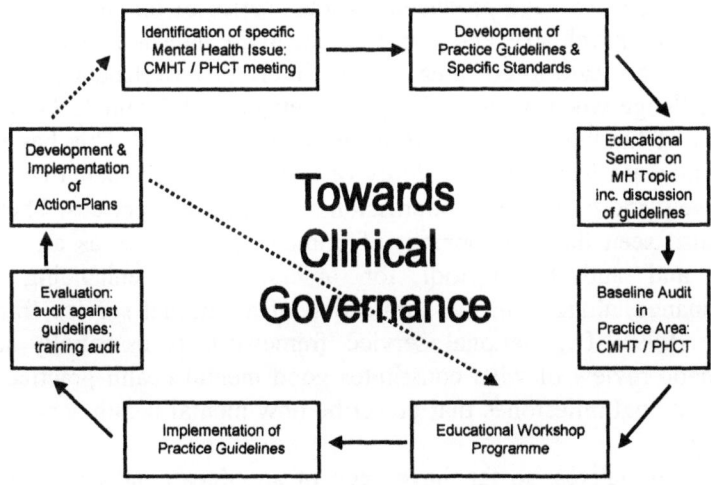

**Figure 13.3 Towards clinical governance**

All these audit and training activities feed into the cycle of clinical governance (see Figure 13.3). Primary care mental health facilitators will have an important part to play in clinical governance across the primary/secondary care interface. Specific issues can be identified through a joint meeting between a PCG and the local CMHT. Specific standards and practice guidelines can be agreed. These guidelines can be established by an educational seminar for the local practices, and baseline audits can be carried out at CMHT and PCT level.

The educational workshop leads on to the implementation of practice guidelines. Subsequently, evaluation of the results of the training can be carried out by further audit, and the action plans deriving from this can lead to identification by the PCG and the CMHTs of further issues. Then, the cycle can be repeated. One hopes that the educational activity with PCGs will enhance GPs' knowledge of modern mental health issues and, therefore, will both enhance primary care practice and PCG commissioning.

## Conclusion

In conclusion, we have produced a robust series of initiatives to improve primary care psychiatry, and joint-working at the interface between primary and secondary care in our area. It was timely that we began to face up to this challenge when we did. The years between 1997 and 1999 have seen the end of fundholding and the development of PCGs. This has meant a major increase in the responsibility of GPs to manage their own services effectively and to begin to commission mental health services. These years have also seen the development of clinical governance, as an evidence-based and audit-based tool for assessing and enhancing clinical performance, along with the publication of a national service framework (DoH, 1999). The national service framework is essentially a major systematic review of what constitutes good mental health practice, with a set of national milestones that prescribe how mental health services are to develop.

The initiatives, so far, have been of an educational nature, but have also included audit activities. It would not have been possible to target the initiatives properly if we had not first developed a model of how all the members of primary care and community mental health teams should work together. As we have adopted a whole system approach to improving primary and secondary mental health care, we still have a great deal of work to do in order to completely modernise mental health services in Bedfordshire. However, substantial progress has been made, and our team was awarded NHS Beacon status in 1999. We look forward now to completing the work begun in 1997 when we started training as mental health facilitators.

## References

Department of Health (1999), *National Service Framework for Mental Health,* Department of Health, London.

Gask, L., Sibbald, B. and Creed, F. (1997), 'Evaluating Models of Working at the Interface Between Mental Health Services and Primary Care', *British Journal of Psychiatry*, vol. 170, pp. 6-11.

Goldberg, D. and Gournay, K. (1997), *The General Practitioner, the Psychiatrist and the Burden of Mental Health Care*, Maudsley Discussion paper No.1, London.

Kessler, D., Lloyd, K., Lewis, G., Pereira Gray, D. (1999), 'Cross Sectional Study of Symptom Attribution and Recognition of Depression and Anxiety in Primary Care', *British Medical Journal,* vol. 318, pp. 436-39.

Mann, A.H., Beizard, R., Murray, J., Smith, J.A., Botega, N., MacDonald, E. and Wilkinson, G. (1998), 'An Evaluation of Practice Nurses Working with General Practitioners to Treat People with Depression', *British Journal of General Practice,* vol. 48, pp. 875-9.

Mynors - Wallace, L., Davies, I., Gray, A., Barbour, F. and Gath, D. (1997), 'A Randomised Controlled Trial and Cost Analysis of Problem-Solving Treatment for Emotional Disorders Given by Community Nurses in Primary Care', *British Journal Psychiatry*, vol. 170, pp. 113-9.

Onyett, S., Pidd, F., Cohen, A. and Peck, E. (1996), 'Mental Health Service Provision and the Primary Care Team', *The Mental Health Review*, vol. 1, pp. 8-16.

Paykel, E.S. and Priest, R.G. (1992), 'Recognition and Management of Depression in General Practice; Consensus Statement', *British Medical Journal*, vol. 305, pp. 1198-1202.

Tylee, A. (1999), 'RCGP Mental Health Management Course', *Journal of Primary Care Mental Health,* vol. 1. pp. 13-4.

# 14 Team Working: From Theory to practice
VIMAL KUMAR SHARMA

## Introduction

The author is a NHS Consultant Psychiatrist and has an interest in developing mental health services in the primary care setting. In the last four years he has led a multi-professional mental health team working alongside primary care teams in Liverpool. Multi-disciplinary team working is central to the successful delivery of mental health services and the targeting of people with severe and enduring mental health problems. This chapter highlights the need, the barriers and the way forward to achieving effective multi-disciplinary team working. The last section of the chapter describes the process of setting up an effective mental health team in a primary care setting in Liverpool.

## Need for Multi-disciplinary Team Working

Multi-disciplinary team working has become a conventional complement of mental health service delivery systems. The most recent documents issued by the Department of Health (DoH, 1997; 1998a; 1998b; 1999a) emphasize the need for an integrated and well-coordinated service and discuss how perennial problems can be overcome. The *National Service Framework for Mental Health* ( DoH, 1999b) has been developed with the assistance of an expert reference group, which brought together health and social care professionals, service users and carers, health and social services managers, and other relevant agencies. Another document, *Modernising Social Services* (DoH, 1998b), highlights difficulties in bringing together different agencies. It states that the government will play a part by removing legal and other obstacles to joint working, and by adopting the same principles, partnership and joint working in policy making as they expect from those who are responsible for delivering the

257

services at local level. The emphasis in this document is on flexible partnership that moves away from sterile conflict over boundaries. Multi-disciplinary team working is necessary for setting priorities; targeting available resources; lessening duplication of work by different professionals; and, providing efficient, integrated and supportive services for the mentally ill (Leathard, 1994).

The failure of care in the community for mentally ill people, arising from poor communication and low morale in professionals, is well-recognised (DoH, 1995). Proper teamwork enables the establishment of a robust communication mechanism. Multi-factorial etiology of mental disorders, ranging from genetic to psychosocial factors, warrants a thorough multi-professional assessment. Teamwork makes it easy to complement each other's assessments and to arrive at a multi-dimensional understanding of mental health problems. Treatment outcome of mental disorders is often superior when drug treatment is combined with psychological and social therapies. A team approach, therefore, helps in complementing different types of treatments given to patients. Proper collaborative working allows a pulling together of the contributions provided by different members of the team in assessment and care planning for patients. This avoids duplication of work. The key worker feels supported by other team members whilst maintaining continuity of care. The team members feel that they are supported by each other, and that in turn raises team morale. Patients and their carers also feel confident in the knowledge that they have the back-up of the whole team for their care. Lastly, working closely together in a team helps in over-coming professional prejudices and fosters inter-professional learning (Parsell and Bligh, 1998). Despite its support in several government documents, progress in inter-professional collaboration has been relatively slow (Roberts and Priest, 1997).

## Barriers to Multi-Disciplinary Team Working

The literature identifies several barriers to multi-disciplinary team working. These may concern: inter-professional issues; primary and secondary care services; clinical and academic issues; management and mental health teams; and, adaptation to change.

- *Inter-Professional Issues*

Inter-professional rivalry, prejudices and leadership conflicts often lead to a dysfunctional team. Lack of clarity of roles and responsibilities often lead to inter-personal conflicts. Traditionally, different professionals have very little exposure to other disciplines during their training. This gives rise to a rather narrow outlook on mental health issues and a focus on a specific model of mental disorder. Exposure to team work may make professionals feel insecure and defensive; they therefore retreat to their own professional shelter.

- *Primary and Secondary Services*

A distinct boundary between primary and secondary care still exists. The reasons for this are linked to their different management structures and different sets of priorities (Kendrick and Hilton, 1997). For example, for GPs 'common mental disorders' remain the area of their main concern, whereas the specialist mental health team is directed to manage severely mentally ill patients. The reality of multi professional team working is that primary and secondary care teams have to work together and set priorities for their patients, depending on their needs.

- *Clinical and Academic Issues*

Teams are expected to apply evidence-based practice. Much work is needed to evaluate various treatment methods, which have proved to be effective in research settings, but have yet to be applied in the real world. Exclusion criteria, refusers and dropouts from a research study exclude many patients. Treatment and management of such patients remain a real challenge for the multi-disciplinary teams. The need for multi-disciplinary work is much talked about, but there is little evidence of its effectiveness (Leathard, 1994).

- *Management and Mental Health Teams*

Managers are often driven by political and economic agendas. They remain under pressure to achieve the targets set out by the Department of Health. As a result they impose policies on mental health teams to be implemented without team members' active involvement. The whole exercise is perceived as unwanted bureaucracy by the team members. Another difficulty is that different professionals are managed by different mangers and organisations. They are often directed by the policies and priorities of their line management. There is still a long way to go to reach a consensus between health and social services in formulating an integrated strategy for delivering mental health services.

- *Adaptation to Change*

Rapid change in the health service, as well as the social welfare system, puts all workers under stress. The source of stress is partly due to lack of adaptability to change. A resistance to change by different team members leads to a lack of cohesiveness in the team.

## The Way Forward for Effective Team Working

Poulton and West (1994) reviewed different models of effective team working in the primary care setting. In the 'Goal Model' the team is concerned about the end product. The 'System Resource Model' measures the team's ability to acquire resources, and the 'Internal Process Model' assesses the team's efficiency and internal processes of problem-solving. The authors conclude that a 'Constituency Approach', in which all the relevant views are incorporated in judging the team's effectiveness, is the most appropriate model for primary health care teams. Vanclay (1998) enumerates components of successful team working in business: i.e. shared goals, well-defined roles, clear procedures, effective communication, mutual support, team members' commitment and regular audit. Moulder *et al.*, (1988) describe difficulties encountered in making their multi-disciplinary team work in a rehabilitation service and the way they resolved them by clarifying professionals' roles, improving communication and setting evaluation procedures.

## Essential Components of Successful Team Working

Consensus about the conceptual basis of mental health care is a particularly important aspect of successful team working in mental health. Munetz *et al.*, (1993) identified the following eighteen basic assumptions that were necessary for the care of severely mentally ill (SMI) people by their multi-disciplinary team:

1.  People with severe mental illness suffer from a real disease;
2.  The expression of the disease is dependent on genetic, personal and environmental factors;
3.  People with SMI have vulnerability to relapse;
4.  They need a thorough multi-dimensional assessment;
5.  The illness has to be distinguished from the person who suffers from the illness;
6.  The treatment and the rehabilitation plans change depending on the phase of illness;
7.  Patients with capacity have the right to decide about their management;
8.  If patients are unaware of their illness they have the right to receive treatment;
9.  They have the right to live independently;
10. Each patient should have an individual care plan;
11. One has to acknowledge that patients have many needs in different areas;
12. Treatment and rehabilitation must occur concurrently;
13. Professionals have to maintain certain boundaries in providing care;
14. Some patients need active and assertive treatment;
15. Their basic needs should be met;
16. Their family and carers must be involved in evaluation, treatment, education and support;
17. All treatments and rehabilitation are collaborative; and,
18. The team has to utilise the findings of good research in their practice.

By accepting these assumptions the team forms a common language in providing care plans.


## Liverpool Primary Care Mental Health Project

In October 1994 Liverpool Health Authority commissioned Aintree Hospital Mental Health Directorate to provide mental health services to a defined population registered with five general practices. A three year project was set up to be monitored through a steering group consisting of purchasers, providers, representatives of GPs, social services, patients' advocacy workers, public health representatives, the University of Liverpool and other relevant agencies. The proposed cost of the project was £150,000 per year, but as part of the reorganisation of services in the directorate, the project team was allocated approximately £200,000 per year to maintain parity with other teams.

The Primary Care Mental Health Project started work in north Liverpool. The remit of this regionally funded project was to:

- establish a community-based multi-disciplinary team, working alongside primary care teams;
- develop a system for primary health care teams in meeting agreed standards for mental health care;
- develop guidelines for agreed referrals, interventions and continuing care within an audit framework between primary and secondary care; and,
- measure performance indicators relevant to national and local priorities.

The team adopted a shared care approach by:

- developing a practice protocol detailing referral procedures, roles and responsibilities of the professionals working with mentally ill patients;
- providing specialists' facilities, such as outpatient clinics, multi-disciplinary team meetings, and assessment clinics run by the community mental health nurses in the primary care setting, with an active involvement of the GPs and other primary care team staff;
- establishing a minimum data-set of the clinical activities within an audit framework;
- holding a practice-based case register of patients with severe mental disorders to improve monitoring of their care through the Care Programme Approach in partnership with the primary care team staff;
- providing certain treatment facilities in the primary care setting, such as depot administration and lithium monitoring;

- co-ordinating services provided by other agencies, such as counselling services, day centres, housing agencies and other voluntary organisations; and,
- enhancing the ability of primary care team staff in dealing effectively with mental health problems by providing training and education.

The aim was also to produce a model for other mental health teams in Liverpool, and to produce a research-based service founded on measured needs and the opinions of service users.

## Primary Care Mental Health Project Team

The Primary Care Mental Health Project team, consisting of a consultant psychiatrist with a trainee, four community mental health nurses (one G grade and three F grades), one client support worker, one carer support worker and one full-time and one part-time secretary, became operational from 1st January 1996. There was funding for a part-time research/audit assistant who was appointed for one year. The team also had input from two social workers from Liverpool District and one social worker from South Sefton District. The Clinical Psychology Department assigned a clinical psychologist who could spare only one session a week for the teamwork. The team had an active contribution from an independent advocacy worker (from MIND). The social workers, psychologist and client advocacy worker were employed and managed by their respective organisations.

The team was based at the purpose-built extension of one of the GP surgeries. Most of the clinical activities, including outpatient consultation and community mental health nurses' assessment and monitoring clinics, were organised in the primary care setting, i.e. at respective general practices.

## Operational Policy and Procedures

An operational policy was formulated after consultation with all the relevant agencies. Our priority was to provide care for severely mentally ill patients. At the same time we agreed to assist primary care teams to deal with common mental health disorders. Our emphasis was to distribute the resources in the most equitable way to all the practices. As far as possible we wished to provide services in the primary care setting. The Steering Group monitored the team's work, meeting every two months.

*Operational Process*

The team adopted a shared care approach whereby members of all the relevant agencies were actively involved in managing patients with mental disorders. The following procedures were implemented to achieve this objective:

• *Referral meetings* Referrals from all sources were pooled together and discussed in the weekly team referral meeting. The patients, depending on their needs, were allocated to the most appropriate professional for an initial assessment. The meetings also gave an opportunity to receive feedback from the mental health professionals following their assessments, as well as to get appropriate advice from team members for a patient's further management.

• *Multi-disciplinary team meetings in the primary care setting* The team organised multi-disciplinary team meetings in the GP practices at their convenience. These were conducted on a rotational basis. The GPs attended most of these meetings. Patients with severe mental disorders were reviewed under the Care Programme Approach, which also provided a forum to discuss other patients with the GPs or team members if they needed any advice or assistance in their management.

## Process of Inter-professional Working

The author and colleagues closely examined the process of inter-professional working in the project team (Sharma *et al.*, forthcoming), and identified the following essential components of successful team working:

• common objectives and goals;
• team involvement in setting up a framework to achieve its objective;
• commitment of the team members;
• clarity of roles and responsibilities;

- clarity of decision-making process and procedures to resolve difficulties;
- set up an audit for periodic evaluation;
- mutual trust and respect;
- shared responsibilities;
- shared success and shared distress;
- adequate support from management;
- common conceptual basis of mental health care; and,
- identification of a team leader.

## The Process of Integrating Services

The Liverpool Primary Care Mental Health Project has demonstrated that a specialist mental health team can be established in general practice; the model of working appears beneficial for patients as well for GPs. This project has given us an opportunity to examine the processes of integrating services between primary and secondary care. In our view the advantages of this model of service delivery outweighed the disadvantages. In the following section we report the difficulties and benefits of this model of service delivery, based on our experiences.

## Difficulties Encountered in the Process of Service Development

Difficulties related to the concerns of both primary health care teams and the mental health team:

- *Primary Care Concerns*

There was a view among primary care reception staff that close working with the mental health team would add to their workload. GPs expressed concern about the administrative and prescription costs involved in providing facilities for mental health professionals in their practices.

- *Mental Health Team Concerns*

The team had concerns about a high volume of demand (especially from people suffering from common mental disorders) from the primary health care teams because of increased accessibility. The high expectations held by the Health Authority of the new team, and the move from a hospital-based to a practice-based system, added to the pressures felt by the team members. As a consequence, this led to a rapid turnover of staff.

It took over 18 months to resolve the staffing difficulties. The team initially had a rapid turnover of community mental health nurses and, on average, did not exceed more than three nurses at any one time. During this time the community mental health nurses began to appreciate the results of close working with the Primary Care Teams. Additionally, GPs and staff saw a distinct advantage for their patients of the new way of service provision.

In the initial phase of our project, professionals with different backgrounds had difficulties in working as a team. The main reason for this was emphasis on different models of care. For example, social workers were against a "medical model" of service delivery. It took over twelve months to establish trust and mutual respect among team members, emphasising a common goal of improved patient care.

## Impact of Multi-disciplinary Mental Health Team Working in a Primary Care Setting

Benefits of the model we adopted were twofold:

- *Efficient Use of Resources*

The efficiency of our use of resources improved by fairer distribution of psychiatrist's time; linking community mental health nurses with the primary care teams; prompt assessment of patients by the most appropriate mental health professional; and, improved communication between primary care teams and mental health professionals. We also managed to reduce the waiting time for new patients. Our team worked closely with the primary care teams to manage patients with both severe mental disorders and common mental disorders. Contrary to the findings of other primary care work (Tyrer, 1984; Goldberg *et al.*, 1996), we didn't find any increase in the number of referrals for common mental disorders. This could have been due to an adherence to the agreed practice protocol that highlighted the use of other community resources for such disorders. The GPs felt more confident in dealing with mentally ill patients, having an easy accessibility to the team members.

- *Effectiveness*

A reduction of over 38% in in-patient bed usage over a three year period, for the urban population served by the mental health team, suggests that this model of service delivery provides early intervention as well as good continuity of care. A similar reduction in in-patient bed usage has been reported by other community studies (Tyrer, 1984, Puri *et al.*, 1996). Improved GP satisfaction with the services also gives indirect indication of the improved effectiveness of our services. High levels of patient satisfaction support the success of this model of service delivery.

## Conclusion

In all parameters of the evaluation the team demonstrated an improvement: i.e. in-patient bed usage; decrease in waiting time for new-patient referrals; increased GP satisfaction with the services; and, improvement in patients' health, social functioning and satisfaction with the services. The team provided a better quality service, by improving continuity and co-ordination of care; training primary health care teams in mental health issues; and, providing services within the primary care setting. The establishment of the team in a primary care setting did not lead to increased demand as originally envisaged.

## References

Department of Health (1995), *Social Services Department and the Care Programme Approach: An Inspection*, Department of Health, London.

Department of Health (1997), *The New NHS: Modern, Dependable*, The Stationery Office, London.

Department of Health (1998a), *A First Class Services – Quality in the New NHS*, Department of Health, London.

Department of Health (1998b), *Modernizing Social Services: Promoting Independence, Improving Protection, Raising Standards*, The Stationery Office, London.

Department of Health (1999a), *Saving Lives: Our Healthier Nation*, The Stationery Office, London.

Department of Health (1999b), *National Service Framework for Mental Health*, Department of Health, London.

Goldberg, D., Jackson, G., Gater, R., Campbell, M., and Jennett, N. (1996), 'The Treatment of Common Mental Disorders by a Community Team Based in

Primary Care: a Cost-Effectiveness Study', *Psychological Medicine,* vol. 26, no, 3, pp. 487-92.

Kendrick, T., and Hilton, S. (1997), 'Primary Care: Opportunities and Threats. Broader Teamwork in Primary Care', *British Medical Journal,* vol. 314, no. 7081, pp. 672-5.

Leathard, A. (1994), 'Inter-Professional Developments in Britain', in A. Leathard (ed), *Going Inter-Professional,* Routledge, London, pp. 3-38.

Moulder, P.A., Stall, A.M. and Grant, M. (1988), 'Making the Inter-Disciplinary Team Aproach Work', *Rehabilitation Nursing,* vol. 13, no. 6, pp. 338-9.

Munetz, R., Birnbaum, A., Wyzik, P. (1993), 'An Integrative Ideology to Guide Community-Based Multi-disciplinary Care of Severely Mentally Ill Patients', *Hospital and Community Psychiatry,* vol. 44, no. 6, pp. 551-5.

Parsell, G. and Bligh, J. (1998), 'Inter-Professional Learning', *Postgraduate Medical Journal,* vol. 74, no. 868, pp. 89-95.

Poulton, B.C., and West, M.A. (1994), 'Primary Health Care Team Effectiveness: Developing a Constituency Approach', *Health and Social Care,* vol. 2, pp. 77-84.

Puri, B.K., Hall, A. D., Reefat, R., Mayer, R., and Tyrer, P. (1996), 'General Practitioners' Views of an Open Referral System to a Community Mental Health Service', *Acta Psychiatric Scandinavica,* vol. 94, no. 2, pp. 133-6.

Roberts, P., Priest, H. (1997), 'Achieving Inter-Professional Working in Mental Health', *Nursing Standard,* vol. 12, no. 2, pp. 39-41.

Sharma, V. K., Wilkinson, G., Dowrick, C., Church, E., White, S. 'Developing Mental Health Services in a Primary Care Setting: Liverpool Primary Care Mental Health Project', *forthcoming.*

Tyrer, P. (1984), 'Psychiatric Clinics in General Practice. An Extension of Community Care', *British Journal of Psychiatry,* vol. 145, pp. 9-14.

Vanclay, L. (1998), 'Teamworking in Primary Care', *Nursing Standard,* vol. 12, no. 20, pp. 37-38.

# 15 Establishing Mental Health Registers in General Practice
ROBIN WILLIAMS

## Introduction

During the early 1990s, community mental health nurses (CPNs) based in Wirral decided to actively negotiate with GP fundholders in order to raise their own profile and aim for greater professional independence, rather than accept the more traditional ways of working, e.g. accepting consultant only referrals. The CPNs became an increasingly potent force in the purchasing arena; many negotiations focused on practices having named CPNs who were practice-attached, running independent psychological clinics. Some fundholders actually refused to sign up with acute provider Trusts until the named individuals were identified.

As a consequence of this process, the author, a trained general and psychiatric nurse, joined St Hilary Brow Group Practice (then a third wave fundholding practice) as a nurse clinician. As part of the process of patient identification, the practice team aimed to establish who the seriously mentally ill were. They developed a comprehensive register for patients with severe and enduring mental illness - an initiative which has led to the team being singled out as an example of good practice in the *National Service Framework for Mental Health* (DoH, 1999). Earlier attempts to identify patients with a diagnosis of schizophrenia across the Wirral (population of 350,000), had identified 800 patients with schizophrenia. However, with the literature indicating a variable incidence of schizophrenia, ranging from 0.13 - 0.69 per 1,000 (Hafner, 1987), the accuracy of local figures was called into question. There appeared to be no formal method of collecting the data. One big advantage of working closely with a well-organised general practice was that it would allow the author to establish in detail the identified number of patients with schizophrenia. The other motivating factor was to take psychiatry away from the institutional arena into a more independent, stigma-free environment. This chapter will describe this process in some detail.

## Background

Since the 1950's general practice has been recognised as the cornerstone for community mental health services (WHO, 1973). Whilst detection of mental illness rates are low and psychiatric morbidity high, only 5% of people recognised as emotionally distressed are referred on to secondary services (Goldberg and Huxley, 1992). Therefore, primary care is well placed to provide an early detection, recognition and treatment service. Attempting to develop a responsive service for people in general practice with minor to more serious forms of mental illness has been an on-going development at the St. Hilary Brow Group Practice since 1992.

    The imaginative fiscal controls allowed under fundholding permitted the employment of staff on a sessional basis. The diversity of skills provided by the staff enabled them to direct their energies towards the patients identified by the practice mental health register. For example, someone suffering with a chronic form of schizophrenia may possess little in the way of social skills and may, therefore, benefit from an improved network of agencies. The occupational therapist has the skills to help such a patient to develop relationships and friendships that are outside mainstream health care. This might involve helping patients to join clubs or gyms, attend training classes, and even become eligible for limited employment. In this way, care and registration have become a symbiotic process, as more comprehensive therapy is available at practice level, which previously might have required secondary care referral. This 'new' style of treatment has the knock-on effect of speeding up access to treatment, which leads to reduced dependency, thus allowing patients to have a fuller and more rewarding life.

    The emphasis, therefore, has been to identify vulnerable patients via the use of a register, and to provide timely and appropriate help from a range of practice-attached staff. The attached staff, all employed by the local Community Trust (see Table 15.1), work closely with the primary care team. The combined team, with extensive input from the GPs, practice nurses and health visitor, work on an internal referral pattern. Once in the 'system,' patients can self-refer to an appropriate member of the team. This reduces bureaucracy, and allows GPs to reduce their 'gatekeeper' role (Horder, 1988), encouraging clinical rather than administrative involvement. This is in contrast to the expected role of a GP.

## Table 15.1  Current mental health team

| ROLE | AREA OF EXPERTISE |
|---|---|
| **Nurse Clinician** (full-time secondment) | Project director; clinical input; co-ordinator of the register |
| **CPN** (one session per week) | Adult mental health CPN; keyworker for Care Programme Approach: provides liaison with local psychiatry department |
| **Consultant Psychologist** (clinic in practice on alternate weeks) | Consultant clinical psychologist; psychosomatic/ Women's health |
| **Counselling** **A.** (one session per week) | Palliative care; bereavement/Relate/trainer for voluntary staff |
| **B.** (one session per week) | Stress/relationship/Family Therapy |
| **C.** (one session per week) | Cognitive Behavioural Therapy/psycho-sexual |
| **CPN (EMI)** (attends monthly reviews) | 'Named' CPN for the elderly; provides clinical input and advice |
| **Social Worker** (attends monthly reviews) | Approved Social Worker; practice liaison/ Referrals to social services |
| **Alcohol Worker** | Practice liaison with Wirral Alcohol Service |
| **Occupational Therapist** (one session per week) | Anxiety management; group, individual and Social Network Therapy |
| **Drug Worker** (clinic every fortnight) | Drug counsellor; managing ex-heroin addicts on methadone maintenance |

**Practice Profile**

The practice has a 5,500 population, and the majority (87%) live within a 2km radius of the practice, which is predominantly urban. The local electoral ward fails to score in terms of health deprivation, e.g. Jarman and Townsend indicators. However, the Super Profiles typology, devised by staff of the University of Liverpool (Batey and Brown, 1995), shows the practice population to have lifestyle groupings at either end of the social spectrum. These indicators allow the practice to compare its own population with the local Wirral population. The practice population is spread across a number of local electoral wards, some of which are very seriously deprived, with high levels of need (see Figures 15.1 and 15.2).

Townsend indicators are used to indicate an overall level of deprivation in a given area. This tends to look at residents who are economically active, own cars and houses, and numbers of people who reside in one room. There is no allowance for social, cultural or other forms of deprivation. Other deprivation indicators, such as Jarman, have a heavy weighting for ethnic minorities (72.5%). Jarman also considers old people living alone, single parent households, children under 5, unskilled people and overcrowded households. In the Mersey region, there is a low prevalence of ethnic minorities (6.3%), so Jarman may not be the most useful of indicators for the local Wirral population.

The Super Profiles neighbourhood types, developed by Batey and Brown (1995) in conjunction with CDMS Ltd., comprise a classification of small areas based upon data derived from the ten-year national census. The typology has a wide range of applications (Batey, Brown and Corver, 1999) and the area types are broadly consistent with the Jarman-Townsend indicators. Their value in measuring the socio-economic status of an area is shown in Figure 15.1. The extremes of the 10 Lifestyle levels of the classification, represented by lifestyles A and J, are described below (CDMS, 1994):

Lifestyle A – Affluent Achievers

High income families with a lifestyle to match. Detached houses predominate, reflecting the professional status of their owners. Typically living in the stockbroker belt of the major cities, members of this group are likely to own two or more cars, which are top of the range, recent purchases and are needed to pursue an active social and family life. People in this neighbourhood type have sophisticated tastes and aspirations. They eat out regularly, go to the theatre and opera and take an active interest in sports (such as, cricket, rugby union and golf). They are able to afford several expensive holidays each year.

Lifestyle J – The 'have nots'

Single parent families, living in cramped, overcrowded flats is the everyday reality of this group which is composed of young adults with large numbers of young children. These are the underprivileged who move frequently in search of a break. However, with two and a half times the national rate of unemployment, and with low qualifications, there seems little hope for the future. Most are on Income Support, and those who can find work are in low paid, unskilled jobs. There are very few cars and little chance of getting away on holidays. Recreation comes mainly from the television and the take up of satellite and cable TV is high. Betting is also popular, particularly on greyhound racing. The Sun and The Mirror are the most popular newspapers.

## Developing a Practice-Based Mental Health Register

The initial drive or idea of creating a mental health register stemmed from a number of thoughts. The *Building Bridges* document proposed that a very broad range of mental illnesses should be registered (DoH, 1995). In reality, this becomes an onerous task which, in practice, we found to be unrealistic and burdensome. Very little information was available in the literature to answer our questions:

- would registers make a difference in terms of changing or altering the venue of care?

- did the practice have a disproportionately large or small number of mentally ill patients?

- would a register change patient care ?

- would it alter the style of care by reducing attendance at hospital, and so admissions and outpatient sessions?

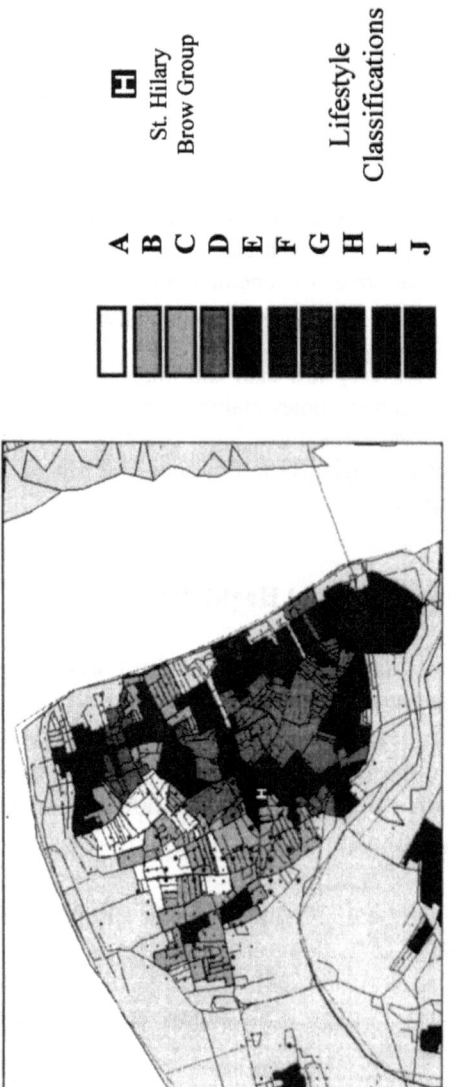

St. Hilary
Brow Group

Lifestyle
Classifications

A
B
C
D
E
F
G
H
I
J

**Figure 15.1  Super-profile classification of practice population**

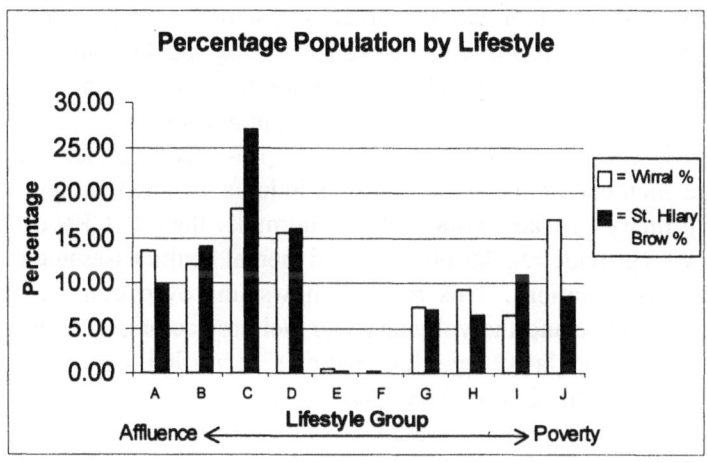

**Figure 15.2 Practice population by lifestyle**

## Methods Adopted in Drawing-up the Register

We started by identifying patients with schizophrenia and manic-depressive psychosis; patients often regarded as traditionally falling out of care, having at one time been hospitalised and possibly suffering the damaging effects of institutionalisation. The group was also recognised as suffering social isolation and poor physical health, and lacking the social confidence to ask for assistance.

Development of the register began by searching the practice drug information computer, looking for all drugs prescribed in the relevant dosage for the treatment of psychotic conditions. For example, low doses of Trifluoperazine were avoided, as this might create a list of people with chronic anxiety states. However, searching for patients treated with Thioridazine, 100mgs or more, created an abundance of patients. Unfortunately, audit of this group of 250 patients revealed a substantial number with agitated dementia and resident in local nursing homes. Other methods that proved most valuable were CPN caseload analysis and neuroleptic home therapy. Figure 15.3 illustrates this in more detail.

Local information from postmen, reception staff etc. provides important feedback about known individuals who are registered at the practice. Some may be behaving in an abnormal way, suggesting mental illness or just eccentricity. This increased level of information, dealt with in a sensitive manner, can only be useful to alert staff of pending problems.

Patients who are registered receive a pro-active service from an appropriate member of the team. This includes a planned review by an identified primary care key worker; this is normally the GP, CPN or Nurse Clinician, who provide regular physical and mental health assessment, with appropriate investigations. This review allows improved communication between the practice and the voluntary and welfare sectors, and secondary care services, particularly regarding patients identified under the Care Programme Approach (CPA) (DoH, 1990).

The initial registration of patients has now been extended to include those suffering chronic depression, defined as someone suffering depression of at least one year's duration. This group remains registered until they have been well and off treatment for one calendar year. We have now also included patients with dementia. This group is identified using a mini-mental state examination with scores less than 25/30 (Folstein, 1975). Patients remain on this part of the register for life.

The initial paper exercise of registration has now been computerised, using a Windows '95 and Access '97 programme, designed, built, tested and networked within the practice. This helps provide instant and speedy retrieval of data, allowing complete automation of the project. We needed to develop something that was dynamic, flexible and capable of interpreting clinical activity and capturing individuals who needed continued support, supervision and monitoring. Attempting to succeed by using paper became a hopeless task. Interrogating paper records is futile, labour intensive and slow. Indeed, the practice personnel had a much clearer idea of who needed care at the most appropriate time than paper was able to reflect or achieve. We felt a computerised register would allow proper evaluation of registers to take place. The local Primary Care Group (PCG) and Health Authority have now decided to adopt our software, which will allow a more comprehensive evaluation of registers to take place since the PCG covers a 70,000 population in over 17 practices. This 'new' electronic approach has the same potential to reduce acute hospital bed occupancy rates as in our own practice. This would amount to 18 fewer beds occupied annually, creating savings of some £250,000.

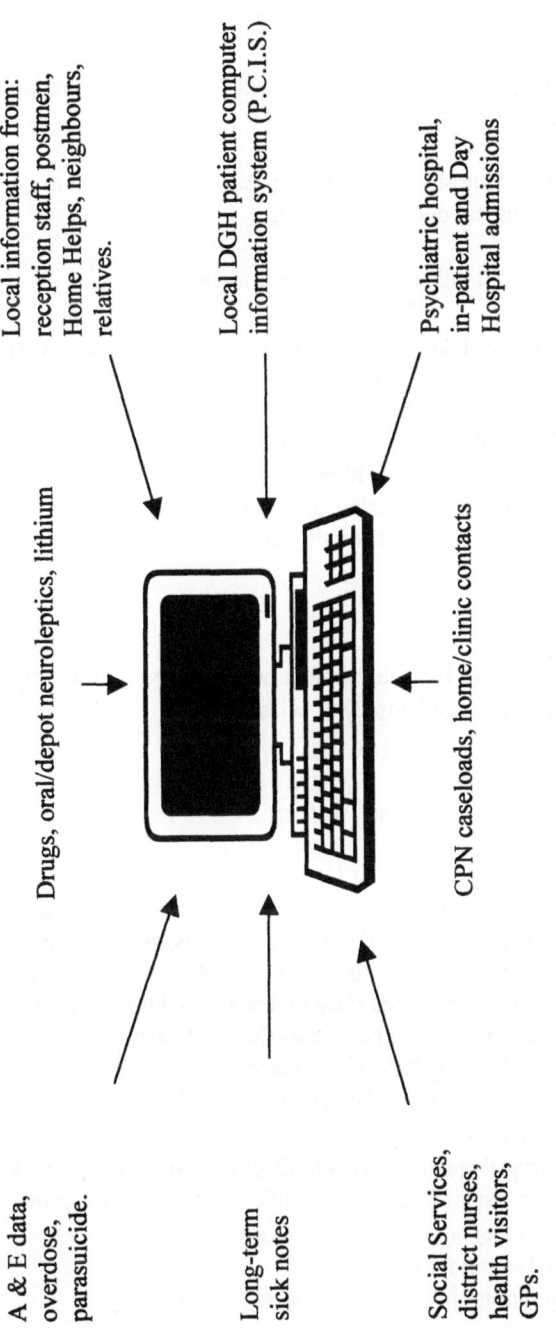

Local information from: reception staff, postmen, Home Helps, neighbours, relatives.

Local DGH patient computer information system (P.C.I.S.)

Psychiatric hospital, in-patient and Day Hospital admissions

Drugs, oral/depot neuroleptics, lithium

CPN caseloads, home/clinic contacts

A & E data, overdose, parasuicide.

Long-term sick notes

Social Services, district nurses, health visitors, GPs.

**Figure 15.3 Creating an electronic mental health register**

*Key Elements of a Mental Health Register*

- password protected; utilises patient consent and empowerment – a proactive approach;

- provides fast, up-to-date, summarised and reliable data. This ultimately improves clinical decision-making;

- duplication of clinical information is avoided;

- sessionally employed clinical staff can share information without the need for face-to-face contact; and,

- whilst the public and professionals have doubts about sharing electronic information, a survey within the practice indicates patients are more concerned about optimising and improving their health care;. concerns about security and confidentiality appear to be a secondary consideration.

*Process of Registration*

Patients are identified by diagnosis and severity. Once registered, basic patient details are recorded together with:

- registered GP;
- identified primary care key worker;
- ICD 10 diagnosis;
- risk assessment in terms of identified and known risks for patients seen at home by professionals. This is displayed as a simple traffic light system: red indicates danger and therefore it is inadvisable for health professionals to visit; amber represents caution with visits only advisable in the company of others; green shows there are no known visiting risks;
- previous treatments are noted together with outpatient attendance and any admissions that may have taken place;
- current and past clinical data are also recorded, together with next of kin;
- CPA details;
- current drug therapy, based on all drugs listed within the BNF (4.0-4.3). Use of drop-down lists help simplify and speed up the process;
- a variety of Reports on patients are available;
- automated reminder letters; and,
- labelling facility for the Lloyd-George notes.

This programme is networked across the practice so the data are instantly available to the entire team at any time.

## Impact of the Mental Health Register

*Patient Satisfaction with Services*

An in-house survey was conducted at the practice. This consisted of 50 randomly selected registered patients, some of whom were quite paranoid. The survey indicated there were no objections to the use of the register. It showed that patients appear to welcome the use of a register, and don't feel stigmatised or consider that their privacy has been invaded. It is now practice policy to inform and discuss with all patients that we intend to put them on the register. Patients appear more interested if we can improve the care and treatment that they receive as a result of using a register, which is in sharp contrast to some published opposition (Sayce and Gorman, 1993).

*Admission Rates*

It appears that the introduction of both the register and team approach into patient mental health care have helped bring about substantial changes in the way patients are managed. For example, on the basis of data collected within the practice, there is an indication that the use of acute hospital beds has changed: when patients are admitted they remain hospitalised for less time. Following admission, the likelihood of being re-admitted is also reduced.

*Drug and Alcohol Abuse*

Detection rates at practice level for patients with SEMI diagnosis appear to compare favourably with other published work (Meltzer *et al.*, 1995), perhaps suggesting that the trawl method is a valid and worthwhile procedure. However, the patients registered for drug dependence are only those who are reformed heroin users, now on maintenance methadone. It would not include the extensive use of substances named in the study conducted by Robins and Regier (1991). The drug dependence register was not intended to capture patients using other substances which were habit-forming and in regular use (*ibid.*).

Again, the registration process did not attempt to capture all patients with alcohol related difficulties, but only those who came forward complaining of, or suffering with, social, domestic or physical impairment. The Meltzer *et al.*, (1995) study relies upon self-assessment at household level; anonymous surveys may draw upon greater honesty amongst the public. This may well explain the low detection rate of alcohol and drug problems seen at practice level.

## Discussion

The published data about mental health registers are somewhat limited. Early published work suggested registers create more work, but primary care staff feel neither equipped to cope with the additional demands to establish registers, nor can they offer the time to fulfil the care that is required by vulnerable patients identified by the register (Hassall and Stilwell, 1977). Surveys investigating GP involvement with long-term mentally ill patients suggest that GPs wish to share the care, but very few have practice policies to cope (Kendrick *et al.*, 1994). In this study, one third of those with serious mental illness had no contact with formal psychiatric services, yet primary care staff were generally unaware of this vulnerable group of patients. More often than not these patients attend general practice for routine and minor ailments - a time when the consultation process can be used to monitor their mental state and the use of a drug therapy (*ibid*). Other studies have suggested that people with a serious mental illness are actually more frequent attenders in primary care than are patients with chronic physical disabilities, such as diabetes and asthma (Nazareth and King, 1992).

The Department of Health and the Royal College of Psychiatrists seem unable to see eye-to-eye over supervision registers. These are different from practice-based mental health registers in that they attempt to identify individuals who are most at risk of committing serious violence, suicide or severe self-neglect. These patients should receive the correct care under the Care Program Approach. Harrison and Bartlett argue that supervision registers place professionals in an untenable position, subject to a duty of care which the patient may not choose, or wish, to comply with

(Harrison and Bartlett, 1994). Mental health registers operated at primary care level are more likely to resemble asthma and diabetes registers. This may reduce the psychiatric stigma and may go some way to closing the gap in health care provision.

The advantage of creating registers can be applied across the clinical field for epidemiological purposes. The term, 'seriously and enduringly mentally ill,' is currently fashionable, but the old phrases 'chronic' or 'burnt out' are still well understood and used. Many may argue that registers should include 'the worried well', as evidence suggests that often emotional problems run a chronic and relapsing course (Bowers, 1997). However, it is our experience that registers which follow current government guidelines (DoH, 1995), using definitions of SEMI based on the dimensions of safety, informal/formal care, diagnosis, disability and duration of illness (SIDDD), will lead to an over-inclusive, cumbersome and impractical register.

Our concern at general practice level was to address the chronic psychotic population, who were, and had become, part of the 'revolving door syndrome'. They were becoming institutionalised with each successive admission, and were receiving a patchy, disorganised and poorly co-ordinated service. The emphasis was, therefore, placed on identifying and registering the vulnerable individuals with a diagnosis of psychosis, chronic depression, and more recently dementia. Routinely collected data tends not to link individuals to statistics. By establishing registers at a local level we can connect individuals and their history to outcome measures. In time this may well help produce morbidity and mortality data, help establish a pattern of contacts with a variety of services and facilities, and come to reflect the requirements of this particular population (Woogh, 1987). Changes in trends, and the introduction of new programs, can then be studied in detail. These systems are considered essential to provide feedback for local health authorities, emerging PCGs, and eventually PCTs. This would allow proper evaluation of registers to take place. The World Health Organisation expert committee has emphasised the need to standardise registers using the *Diagnostic Statistical Manual (Issue 3)* (DSM3) and the *International Classification of Diseases (9th and 10th edition)* (ICD9/10), (WHO, 1973; 1992). This helps to improve the reliability of case registers.

Epidemiological studies based on record linkage cannot alone assess treated illness. However, the introduction of computers and general computerisation into general practice allows more complex data to be handled and analysed. Unfortunately, there is a counter-productive effect that can take place: increasing quality also increases the cost and difficulty of data collection.

If we are able to normalise treatment of mental illness at primary care level, patients will need to receive a more rapid and orderly, responsive service. The gap which exists may occur because some professionals do not feel adequately skilled (only 29% of GPs have formal psychiatric training), or do not have personnel to call upon who can complement primary care service provision. The use of a register will highlight and identify vulnerable individuals who fall into the gap. The gap may exist because primary and secondary care fail to communicate. Networked and shared electronics provide an instant means of communication. Nevertheless, some GPs may feel psychiatric responsibility lies with others, i.e. traditional secondary care. Further, the identified workload which registers create may be off-putting, as there are not always sufficient staff in primary care to provide the therapy and support that is required.

## Conclusion

Home-based care by experienced teams is a well-recognised service, which is preferred by patients and carers and is as effective as hospital care (Marks, 1992). Pioneering new styles of care within the NHS is not always clear-cut and straightforward. The NHS, in the guise of health authorities, has historically supported failing general practices by increasing financial assistance. A more pragmatic approach might be to support thriving initiatives in primary care which demonstrate improved health outcomes, for otherwise the less attractive areas of health care may end up suffering most. Mental health is no exception to this formula, and is often seen by GPs as a problem of under-funding. Improved health care is really about imaginative use of existing resources. Instituting care at primary care level is inexpensive (see Table 15.2), and our preliminary evidence suggests it is associated with a favourable change in secondary care service use. This also leads to greater treatment compliance and improved attendance rates.

**Table 15.2 Costs of providing mental health care at primary care level: St Hilary Brow psychiatry budget 1996/7**

| Consultant Psychiatrist | = £ 6,400 | OPD @ £24/case Cost/case follow up from admissions | = £ 400 |
|---|---|---|---|
| CPN | = £ 3,300 | 1 session per week | = £ 3,100 |
| Occupational Therapist | = £ 400 | 1 session per week | = £ 1,400 |
| Psychologist | = £ 1,800 | 1 session fortnightly | = £ 2,400 |
| | | Counselling x13 hours per week | = £ 4,800 |
| **BUDGET** | **= £ 11,900** | **EXPENDITURE** | **= £12,100** |

Rapid access to a wide range of professionals leads to low 'did not attend' (DNA) rates of less than 5%; the traditional secondary care outpatient clinics have DNA rates of 20% for new cases and 30% for repeats. Patients realistically argue the case that there is no continuity of care in secondary care OPD clinics, as they may end up seeing junior hospital doctors on a 6-month training scheme. (Beerforth *et al.*, 1990).

The cross-referral pattern at practice level further reduces bureaucracy and unnecessary paper work. The process also lessens the need for high capital bed cost services, which are less popular with patients and carers. The emphasis is thereby placed on an assertive home care model. Many GPs argue that this is not standard general practice. Through the potency and negotiations which fundholding allowed, personnel were purchased on a sessional basis (see Table 15.1). With the dissolution of fundholding, and the introduction of personal medical services, there was some pressure on the practice to downsize rather than maintain an existing level of staff who could provide quality of care. In some areas of Britain this downsizing has already begun and health authorities have decided not to purchase some services, such as counselling. There is a danger that this will lead to detrimental effects on primary health care provision.

## Acknowledgements

Many thanks to the following individuals who have made valuable and constructive comments about the chapter: Dr. Derek Chiswick, Consultant Forensic Psychiatrist, Royal Edinburgh Hospital, Edinburgh, Scotland; Dr. Trevor Gibbs, Department of Primary Care, Liverpool University, Liverpool; Sarah Moore, Statistician, Clinical Practice Research Unit, Arrowe Park Hospital, Wirral; Dominic Wilcocks, Information Technology Adviser, St. Hilary Brow Group Practice, Wirral; and, Professor Greg Wilkinson, Royal Liverpool University Hospital, Liverpool.

## References

Batey, P.W.J. and Brown, P.J.B. (1995), 'From Human Ecology to Customer Targeting: the Evolution of Geodemographics', in P. Longley and G. Clarke (eds), *GIS for Business and Service Planning*, Longman, London, pp. 77-103.

Batey, P.W.J, Brown, P.J.B. and Corver, M. (1999), 'Participation in Higher Education: A Geodemographic Perspective on the Potential for Further Expansion in Student Numbers', *Journal of Geographic Systems*, vol. 1, pp. 277-303.

Beerforth, M., Conlon, E., Field, V., Hosher, B. and Sayce, E. (eds) (1990), *Whose Service Is It Anyway? Users Views on Co-ordinated Community Care*, Research and Development in Psychiatry, London.

Bowers, L. (1997), 'Community Psychiatric Nurse Caseloads and the 'Worried Well': Misspent Time or Vital Work?', *Journal of Advanced Nursing*, vol. 26, pp. 930-6.

CDMS (1994), *Super Profiles*, Promotional Brochure produced by CDMS Limited, Liverpool.

Department of Health (DoH) (1990), *Health and Social Services Development: "Caring for People" The Care Programme Approach for People with a Mental Illness referred to the Special Psychiatric Services*, Joint Health and Social Services Circular, HC(90)23LASSL(90)11, Department of Health, London.

Department of Health (DoH) (1995), *The Health of the Nation. Building Bridges: A Guide to Arrangements for Inter-Agency Working for the Care and Protection of Severely Mentally Ill People*, HMSO, London.

Department of Health (1999) (DoH), *A National Service Framework for Mental Health*, Department of Health, London.

Folstein, M. (1975), 'Mini Mental State Examination', *Journal of Psychiatric Research*, vol. 12, pp. 189-98.

Ford, R., Durcan, G. and Warner, L. (1998), 'One Day Survey by the Mental Health Act Commission of Acute Adult Psychiatric Inpatient Wards in England and Wales', *British Medical Journal*, vol. 317, pp. 1279-83.

Goldberg, D. and Huxley, P. (1992), 'Filters in the Pathway to Care', in D. Goldberg and P. Huxley (eds), *Common Mental Disorders: A Biosocial Model*, Tavistock/Routledge, London.

Hafner, H. (1987), 'Epidemiology of Schizophrenia', in H. Hafner, W.F. Gattaz, and W.Janzarik (eds), *In Search for the Causes of Schizophrenia*, Springer-Verlag, Berlin, pp. 47-74.

Harrison, G. and Bartlett, P. (1994), 'Supervision Registers for Mentally Ill People', *British Medical Journal*, vol. 309, pp. 551-2.

Hassall, C. and Stilwell, A. (1977), 'Family Doctor Support for Patients on a Psychiatric Case Register', *Journal of the Royal College of General Practitioners*, October, pp. 605-8.

Horder, J. (1988), 'Working with General Practitioners', *British Journal of Psychiatry*, vol. 153, pp. 513-21.

Kendrick, T., Burns, T., Freeling. P. and Sibbald, B. (1994), 'Provision of Care to General Practice Patients with Disabling Long-Term Mental Illness: A Survey With 16 Practices', *British Journal of General Practice*, vol. 44, pp. 301-305.

Marks, I. (1992), 'Innovations in Mental Health Care Delivery', *British Journal of Psychiatry*, vol. 160, pp. 589-97.

Meltzer, H., Gill, B., Petticrew, M. and Hinds, K. (1995), *The Prevalence of Psychiatric Morbidity Among Adults Living in Private Households*, O.P.C.S., London.

Nazareth, I. and King, M. (1992), 'Schizophrenia: Community Care and the Family Physician', *International Review of Psychiatry*, vol. 4, pp. 267-72.

Robins, L.N. and Regier, D.A. (eds). (1991), *Psychiatric Disorders in America: the Epidemiological Catchment Area Study*, The Free Press (Macmillan Inc.), New York.

Sayce, E. and Gorman, J. (1993), *Mind's Policy on Case Registers*, MIND, London.

Woogh, C.M. (Aug 1987), 'The Case for Psychiatric Record Linkage', *Canadian Journal of Psychiatry*, vol. 32, pp. 470-5.

World Health Organisation (WHO), (1973), *Psychiatry and Primary Medical Care*, World Health Organisation, Copenhagen.

World Health Organisation (WHO), (1992), *International Classification of Diseases: 10th Revision. Classification of Mental and Behavioural Disorders*, World Health organisation, Geneva.

# 16 Assessing and Managing Risk in People with Severe Mental Illness

JOHN BUTLER AND GARY LEES

## Introduction

To effectively manage risk in the community, national mental health policy has focused attention on targeting people with severe mental illness. Risk assessment and risk management are central to this enterprise. This chapter describes a practical guide for community mental health workers, developed by the authors during their involvement in the 'South Bedfordshire Initiative'. The authors are currently working as Lead Community Mental Health Nurses working within acute, adult mental health. One of the authors (JB) was also the principle author of the local Trust's Community Care Policy. Both are involved in providing an on-going programme of in-service training on risk assessment and risk management to mental health nurses in the Bedfordshire area.

The chapter begins with some background information about risk and mental illness, and the increasing attention given to risk assessment and management. Next, the definition of risk is discussed in relation to the present context of providing mental health care to individuals in the least restrictive environment. A practical method for the assessment of risk is then presented, based upon the development of client risk profiles. This is followed by a discussion of the key principles of formal risk management from the perspective of the community mental health worker, illustrated by client case material taken from the direct clinical experiences of the authors. The chapter is concluded with a discussion of the problems and tensions evident within clinical risk management.

## Background

Over the last thirty years, care for people with mental illness has increasingly moved away from institutions and into community settings. As a result, professionals are faced with new challenges in effectively managing the risks presented by people with severe mental illness living in the community.

It is well known, and becoming increasingly accepted, that only a few people with mental illness people pose real risks to themselves or others (Alberg *et al.*, 1996). In terms of risk:

- an American study estimated that 92% of people with a mental disorder are not violent Swanson *et al.* (1990);
- the risk for suicide or self-harm amongst people with mental illness is much greater than the risk of inflicting harm on others - up to 100 times greater for schizophrenia, and up to 1,000 times greater for affective disorders (Alberg *et al.*, 1996);
- studies of in-patient violence suggest that it is only a small number of patients who are accountable for the majority of violent acts (Crichton, 1995), with various socio-demographic factors being associated with violence: youth, being male, ethnicity, and low socio-economic status (Crichton, 1995; Tardiff and Sweillam, 1980);
- only a small number of patients account for the significant amount of direct observation in acute mental health in-patient settings; and,
- nurses, junior doctors and psychiatrists are able to predict violence with a reasonably high level of accuracy (60%), enhanced by conducting formal risk assessment rather than leaving to chance or intuition alone Lidz *et al.* (1993).

Risk assessment and risk management have gradually become more topical with the publication of a growing number of influential reports based upon numerous inquiries into serious incidents. There have been over 100 in the last 30 years. The recommendations of these reports have, in many cases, still to be fully addressed by specialist services. Most of these highly publicised reports relate to homicides by people with mental illness. They invariably highlight deficiencies in both risk assessment and risk management, and especially relate to the lack of effective communication.

Lipsedge and Bland (1997, p. 171) provide a useful review of the findings of 11 such inquiries into homicides, published between 1995 and 1997. This highlights a series of: 'recurrent topics and themes that may be of interest... to ensure adequate assessment and management of risk'. These findings have consistently been reinforced by other inquiries:

- the need to ensure that vital information is obtained, heeded and passed on to all involved parties, with risk assessment and risk management being conducted by the multi-disciplinary team, involving the consultant psychiatrist (Ritchie *et al.*, 1994, p. 110);
- the need for an adequate appreciation of the client's past history based upon full, detailed and authoritative information, which will be aided by all professional staff remaining familiar with the indicators of risk and risk management options (Main *et al.*, 1996, p.33);
- the over-riding duty to breach confidentiality and to provide information to the extent of being in the interests of a potential victim, if there is a clear risk to a member of the public (Blom-Cooper *et al.*, 1995, p.149);
- the need to involve, listen to and respond to the needs of carers;
- the need for adequate resources - medical staffing, community mental health nurses (CMHNs), social workers, and access to in-patient beds;
- the need for accurate and effective interpretation of the Mental Health Act 1983 (House of Commons, 1983), especially section 117 and sections covering detention and provision for leave;
- the need to assess the client in the community if s/he is refusing or unable to attend an appointment, with the process of risk assessment being continual via face to face reviews by clinicians (Mishcon *et al.*, 1996, p.72).

In addition to the above, it has been concluded that:

- the first referral or transfer of a patient to another team should always lead to a new clinical assessment, incorporating a risk assessment (Blom-Cooper *et al.*, 1995, p. 177);
- risk assessment should be viewed as an essential and integral part of the Care Programme Approach (CPA) (Ealing, Hammersmith and Hounslow Health Authority, 1996, p. 32);
- a case must never be disclosed, nor a patient discharged from mental health care unless the team has detailed, reliable and reassuring information about the patient's current health and welfare, and all requirements under section 117 and the CPA have been fulfilled (Lipsedge and Bland, 1997); and,
- the development of a risk management strategy aimed at promoting the safety and security of patients, staff and the public, will need to incorporate effective communication systems, environmental assessment,

an incident reporting and review system, and a continuing programme of staff training.

More recently, the *National Service Framework for Mental Health* (DoH, 1999) has emphasised:

- the need for formal risk assessment and risk management in providing effective care for people with SEMI (*ibid.*, Standards 4 and 5, pp. 41-51); and,
- the need for health and social services to collaborate in achieving a reduction in the suicide rate by at least one fifth by 2010 (*ibid.*, Standard 7, pp. 76-8).

**Defining Risk**

Risk may be viewed as the possibility and likelihood of beneficial and harmful outcomes occurring within a stated time scale (Alberg *et al.*, 1996, p. 9). This process of assessing the likelihood, or probability of, various harms and benefits occurring may be illustrated in the scenario of granting leave to an in-patient. This may result in the patient not returning to hospital and carrying out further high-risk behaviour. Alternatively, it may lead to increased trust, and hence compliance or collaboration within his or her own treatment.

Risk is a dynamic, ever-changing characteristic, perhaps best considered on a continuum ranging from low risk to high risk. The individual will present varying types and levels of risk as an inevitable consequence of life experiences, thus moving along this risk continuum. This contrasts with the term 'dangerousness', which continues to be widely used within the literature, particularly with respect to people with mental illness who are violent. The term 'dangerous' is used to refer to an individual's capacity to cause serious physical injury or lasting psychological harm. The individual is more likely to be viewed in a categorical way: as dangerous or not dangerous. It is, therefore, argued that risk is likely to be a much more useful concept.

In health care settings, a systematic and objective approach to assessment is needed, due to individual differences based upon values and beliefs. The focus is on probability rather than certainty (Prins, 1981). Risk assessment may be viewed as the approach by which those individuals who present medium or high-risk behaviours are identified. Risk management may be viewed as the approach by which a range of actions and factors, likely to minimise the occurrence and likelihood of assessed risks, are identified and implemented. Risk assessment and risk management thus form an integrated process, which will need to be undertaken on an on-going basis. It will not always be possible to predict and prevent risk behaviour by people with mental illness, as risk assessment is based upon clinical judgement and cannot guarantee accurate predictions.

Four principle categories of harmful risks are frequently cited within the literature:

- violence and aggression;
- suicide and deliberate self-harm;
- severe self-neglect; and,
- risk to children.

We will take each of these in turn:

## Violence and Aggression

Although often used interchangeably, these terms refer to different behaviours and intentions: an individual can behave aggressively without being violent. Aggression is a feeling or action that is hostile or self-assertive by intent; whereas, violence refers to behaviour that results in injury to persons or damage to property (Alberg *et al.*, 1996, p.10).

## Suicide and Deliberate Self-Harm

Suicide and deliberate self-harm may be viewed as falling on a continuum with a number of stages (McLaughlin, 1993). Eldrid (1988) suggests that these include:

- the 'early warning stage' - the active expression of thoughts, feelings and plans of suicide;
- parasuicide - defined as 'the non-fatal act of self-injury or the taking of substances in excess of the generally recognised or prescribed therapeutic dose' (Kreitman, 1987);
- deliberate self-harm - this involves the criterion of committing a deliberate act which the individual knows will harm, but without the intent to die (Morgan, 1979);

- attempted suicide - this refers to a deliberate effort to end one's life, that may have accidentally failed; and,
- suicide - defined as 'the intentional act of self-destruction committed by someone knowing what he is doing and knowing the probable consequences of his action' (Kreitman, 1987).

## Severe Self-Neglect

The assessment of this type of harmful risk is less straightforward, as it is complicated by differences in relative standards of what constitutes self-neglect. Alberg *et al.,* (1996) suggest that factors such as hygiene, diet, infestation, household safety, warmth and physical health should be considered as the principle areas for assessment, as each can become life threatening. Deterioration of the domestic environment, or personal care, may be an indicative sign of deterioration in the individual's mental state.

## Risk to Children

Many mentally ill people are also parents and, as such, may present certain risks to children as a consequence of potentially impaired parenting abilities. The types and levels of risk presented are likely to vary in accordance with the nature, severity and chronicity of the parent's mental health problem. Rates of mental disorder in cases of child homicide are high – 75% (Campion *et al.,* 1988) to 100% (Bourget and Bradford, 1990) of parental perpetrators have been diagnosed as suffering from a major mental illness. As with the afore-mentioned risks, the level of risk presented may vary from minimal to severe neglect, whether emotional, physical or sexual in nature.

## Types of Information and Tools Used in Risk Assessment

### Actuarial Data

This consists of factors that increase the risk of a negative outcome. For example, a man is more likely to become violent than is a woman is, and being depressed increases the chance of suicide. It is important to note that, with this form of data, the best single predictor is only about 30% accurate, and this usually involves having a past history of the risk behaviour. If a range of factors is taken into account, the accuracy can be increased.

*Anamnestic Data*

This refers to data relating to how a person behaved in the past in similar circumstances, and is of greater predictive value than actuarial data. These kind of data are frequently gathered from a clinical interview with the client, but a well informed assessment process should include obtaining information from other sources, such as from relatives or other agencies.

*Clinical Interview*

By use of an interview, it is possible to obtain information from the client that will add depth and meaning to the bare facts of the risk(s) presented. A framework for such an interview is presented later in this chapter. The clinical interview can, and should be, repeated with significant others, such as other professionals, in order to obtain additional information and to corroborate the statement from the client.

*Risk Factors*

Whilst personal and social factors which are known to be associated with violence or suicide are not necessarily causal, their presence does assist in the overall evaluation of a person's level of risk in the long-term. Considering the two principle risk categories of violence and suicide, the major factors associated with an increased risk are summarised in Tables 16.1 and 16.2. The following list of factors pertaining to immediate risk of violence or harm to others, and Table 16.1, draw especially on the work of Alberg *et al.* (1996, p.42), Borum (1996), Lipsedge and Bland (1997, p.174), and Kemshall (1999).

*Indicators of Immediate Risk of Violence or Aggression*

- speaking loudly;
- pacing about;
- easily evoked startle response;
- hyper-vigilance and attentiveness;
- clenched fists; and,
- sitting on edge of seat.

**Table 16.1    Violence or harm to others**

| Variables | Higher Risk |
|---|---|
| Age | Younger |
| Sex | Male (if no psychotic features) |
| Living arrangements | Unstable / changeable / access or proximity to past or potential victims |
| Intelligence | Low |
| Employment status | Unemployed / casual / changeable. |
| Educational attainment | Low |
| Environmental factors | Hot weather / periods of social unrest / life experience in a sub-culture condoning or expecting the use of violence; |
| Physical health | Organic brain disorders; |
| Mental health | Mental illness, especially psychotic Depression / bipolar disorder / schizophrenia with uncontrolled symptoms (a better predictor than past history for people with schizophrenia) / paranoid psychosis / anti-social personality disorder / a history of childhood abuse; |
| Mental health symptoms | Command hallucinations (if there is an history of acting on them) / delusions (passivity, religious, paranormal or physical influence, persecution) / thought insertion / paranoid states; |
| History of violence / aggression | Has an history of aggression or violence (even if this did not result in injury, or was merely a series of repeated minor assaults which have escalated in |

seriousness, but not led to a conviction) - especially the case if the person has a definite plan, and the availability of, and preparedness to use, a weapon;

Forensic history          Has a forensic history involving violence or aggression;

Substance use          Alcoholism; illicit drug use;

Time of week          Saturday.

Table 16.2 and the following list concerning immediate risk in relation to suicide and self-harm, draw especially on the work of Alberg *et al.* (1996), Appleby *et al.* (1999), Clark and Fawcett (1992), Fairlie and Butler (1994), Hawton (1987), Hawton and Fagg (1988), Kreitman (1977), Kreitman and Dyer (1980), McClure (1984), Sainsbury (1955), Schneidman (1976), Tuckman and Youngman (1963; 1968), and Whitlock (1973).

**Table 16.2     Suicide or harm to self**

| Variable | Higher Risk |
|---|---|
| Age | Older and young males; |
| Sex | Male; |
| Marital status | Separated / divorced / widowed / single; |
| Living arrangements | Living alone (social isolation) / absence of children under 18 years old at home / absence of friendships; |
| Employment status | Unemployed / retired; |
| Socio-economic group | High or low socio-economic groups; |

| | |
|---|---|
| Family history | History of affective disorder / alcoholism or suicide in the family; |
| Physical health | Poor (especially terminal, painful, debilitating illness); |
| Mental health | Mental illness (especially depression and if 1-3 lifetime episodes of depression) / schizophrenia / chronic sleep disorders / personality disorder / dual diagnosis; |
| Mental health symptoms | Severe hopelessness / impaired concentration / severe anhedonia / severe anxiety / obsessive-compulsive features / indecisiveness / insomnia / suicidal ideation / pessimistic outlook / periods of clinical improvement following relapse / poor compliance with treatment; |
| History of self-harm / suicide attempts | Has a history of deliberate self-harm or suicide attempt (especially if made in the last year) / by a violent or lethal method e.g. hanging / leaving a suicide note / a definite plan; |
| Significant life events | Bereavement (especially in childhood) / breakdown of intimate relationship; |
| Forensic history | Has a forensic history / imprisonment (especially in the first 24 hours); |
| Substance use | Alcoholism / illegal drug use; |
| Time of year | April to June. |

## *Indicators of Immediate Risk of Suicide or Self-Harm*

- expresses feelings of severe hopelessness;
- expresses suicidal thoughts;
- has a definite plan for suicide;
- has chosen a violent / lethal method for suicide;
- has access to the means to commit suicide;
- makes efforts to maintain privacy for suicide attempt;
- perceives stress as over-whelming, circumstances as unchangeable;
- lack of social supports; and,
- refusal to seek or accept help/ treatment.

## Local Study of Risk Factors in Bedfordshire

In a local audit study (Fairlie and Butler, 1994) of the coroners' records of suicides for 1991-2 in Bedfordshire (N=82), the following patterns were noted:

- the highest risk age-group was 30-39 years old;
- the ratio of male to female suicides was 2.6 : 1;
- in 51% of suicides marital status was divorced, widowed or single;
- in 34% of suicides employment status was unemployed or retired;
- the most common precipitants, recorded for 57 out of 82 suicides, were:
  - breakdown of an intimate relationship (36% - especially if under 45 years of age);
  - financial problems (18%);
  - physical disability and ill-health (13% - especially if under 45 years of age);
  - bereavement (13% - especially if over the age of 45 years);
- females were more likely than males to have made previous attempts;
- 34% of males and 83% of females had a psychiatric diagnosis, with depression being the most common diagnostic category (73% of those with a diagnosis);
- the most common method of suicide for males was vehicle exhaust gas (55%), and hanging (17%); and, for females, drug overdose (33%); and,
- 42% of suicides left a suicide note, a large majority of which appeared to help explain the reasons for suicide.

## The Role of Hopelessness

Much research suggests that a feeling of hopelessness is central to an individual's decision to commit suicide. It appears to be both a concomitant of depression and a predictor of suicidal behaviour (Beck, 1967; 1986). It has been found to predict eventual suicide among individuals diagnosed with a major affective disorder, schizophrenia and alcohol abuse (Beck *et al.*, 1976). Moreover, it seems to distinguish between suicidal and non-suicidal persons with the same level of depression. Hopelessness appears to be a strong predictor of suicide among persons who have made a prior suicide attempt (Dyer and Kreitman, 1984). Longitudinal studies have also shown hopelessness to be a useful long-term predictor of completed suicide. From the above, it appears that a measure of hopelessness is an essential part of any assessment of suicidal intent. Whilst this can be obtained by asking the client how they feel about the future, assessment-rating scales are useful, e.g. the *Beck Depression Inventory* (BDI – Beck *et al.*, 1961) and the *Beck Hopelessness Scale* (BHS – Beck *et al.*, 1974).

*Assessment Rating Instruments*

A number of specialised tools have been developed to complement the assessment process in assisting the clinician to systematically evaluate and determine the seriousness of the risk posed by an individual. It is thus recognised as good practice that risk assessment is supported via the use of formal validated risk assessment schedules. A variety of good examples are available such as the *HCR-20 - Historical and Clinical Risk* (Webster *et al.*, 1995); the *Beck Hopelessness Scale* (Beck *et al.*, 1974; Beck and Steer, 1988); and, the *Beck Scale for Suicide Ideation* (Beck *et al.*, 1988). Borum (1996) presents a useful review of those instruments for assessing violence.

**Guide for Risk Assessment**

It is very useful to make reference to a guide for risk assessment when conducting the clinical interview. Steadman *et al.*, (1994) produced a guide for assessing the risk of violence, suggesting that a number of variables be considered when undertaking an assessment, in order to make 'more accurate, empirically based predictions of risk' (Borum, 1996, p. 947). This guide highlights four sets of factors, which would also have a useful application for the other principle categories of risk:

- dispositional - demographics, personality and cognitive variables;
- historical - family, occupational, psychiatric and forensic history;
- contextual - perceived levels of, and response to, stress, social supports and access to the means for violence or self-harm; and,
- clinical - symptoms, diagnosis and level of functioning.

It is recommended that information is gathered from all available sources, including both formal and informal carers, by several methods of inquiry including interviewing, observation; and data-collection from records and significant others. When assessing and rating risk, Alberg *et al.*, (1996, pp. 42-4; 53-4) recommend that the following are always taken into consideration: risk factors, history of risk, recency, severity, frequency, pattern or context, ideation, plan, and, intent. When considering the patient's history of risk, account should be taken of: relevant incidents in the past and any problems in the past year; the threat of violence or harm, whether verbal or non-verbal; and reports by others of fears for the safety of themselves or others.

When assessing risk, the use of direct questions is recommended. For example, in the case of deliberate self-poisoning or self-injury Hawton and Catalan (1987) suggest the following questions:

- what is the explanation for the attempt in terms of the likely reasons and goals?
- what was the degree of suicidal intent?
- Is the patient at risk of suicide now, or is there an immediate risk of further overdose or self-injury?
- what problems, both acute and chronic, confront the patient?
- did a particular event precipitate the attempt?
- is the patient psychiatrically ill and, if so, what is the diagnosis and how is this relevant to the attempt?
- what kind of help would be appropriate, and is the patient willing to accept such help?

## The South Bedfordshire Initiative

In the South Bedfordshire Community Healthcare Trust, the aims of risk assessment and risk management are to:

- correctly identify the patient who presents medium or high risk behaviours, which fall along a continuum of risk from low to high;
- alert professionals and informal carers of the factors which are likely to increase the level of risk;
- identify and implement factors and actions that are likely to minimise the assessed risks; and
- support the discharge from care of those who have genuinely sustained progress, reinforcing the notion of movement along the 'risk continuum' (South Bedfordshire Community Healthcare Trust, 1998, p.12).

Risk assessment may best be summarised by considering the question: 'Might this patient, in certain circumstances, behave in a way(s) which is dangerous, or of risk to him or herself, or to others?' The clinician is then advised to consider the nature, seriousness and likelihood of all feared outcomes: 'What exactly do I fear this patient might do, when might s/he do it, and to whom?' Framing the risk analysis in this way can help indicate the specific actions required to minimise the level of risk.

Within the Trust, this risk profiling process is closely based upon the tool developed by the Centre for Clinical Outcomes, Research and Effectiveness (British Psychological Society, 1997a): a modified version of this has been described within the Trust's Community Care Policy (South Bedfordshire Community Healthcare Trust, 1998, pp.12-13; 38-40; section 5.3; appendix 8). The risk profile does not dictate the way in which the assessment is carried out, this being left to the professional's discretion. However, joint assessment by two clinicians is recommended as best practice i.e. a named-nurse and CMHT member, or two CMHT members (*ibid*). Rather than being designed as a structured clinical interview, the items covered within the risk profile serve only as an 'aid memoire', or set of checklists, in relation to the history and recency of defined risk behaviours. The profile is used only to record information which is collected through reasonable and practical inquiry, that is, the inspection of any available letter of referral or case notes; the completion of a sensitive clinical interview with the patient and significant others.

For all patients who are subject to the higher categories of the CPA, and all those for whom one or more positive responses are given in an initial 6-item brief risk profile, the multi-disciplinary team is required to carry out and record a full risk profile. This is done through the named-nurse or key-worker, and preferably one other team-member. Particular attention is given to the following major risk types: violence, suicide or attempted suicide, self-harm, self-neglect, capacity for abuse by others, offending behaviours, substance misuse, and risk to children. It is accepted that the patient's level of risk is likely to change in accordance with the following factors: mental state, untoward events, incidents, compliance with treatments, and response to treatments (i.e. medication, psychotherapeutic approaches). Thus, risk assessment will need to be an ongoing process.

Following the completion of the full risk profile, the multi-disciplinary team discusses risk management options. It is recognised that all these will be based upon clinical judgement, with the selected option being the one that is most likely to address the identified risks. Required care interventions should be consistent with the following key principle of being the least restrictive intervention necessary for risk minimisation, as judged against the assessed level of risk, including harm to self, harm to others, and abuse by others. The formal, three-part full risk profile incorporates:

- current warning signs (Risk Profile I and II);
- risk history (Risk Profile I and II);
- feared outcome(s) (Risk Profile II);
- factors likely to minimise risk, with an action decision and rationale (Risk Profile II); and,
- relapse and risk management plan (Risk Profile III) (see British Psychological Society, 1997b; South Bedfordshire Community Healthcare Trust, 1998).

The risk profile is commonly completed following the initial assessment of a new patient or client by the Community Mental Health Team. It may also be completed either upon admission to, or discharge from, an in-patient setting - especially where a succinct summary of risk factors and/or a clear risk management plan is required to be followed upon the patient's discharge. The risk profile is also reviewed at the times of formal CPA review meetings, or at times of significant change in the patient's condition (*ibid.*, p. 13).

*Developing the Relapse and Risk Management Plan*

The final and most important part of the risk profile is designed to summarise the steps to be taken in the event of relapse, signs of relapse, to minimise risk, risk being identified or risk being suspected. Ideally, the relapse and risk management plan is completed with the patient, following discussion with the multi-disciplinary team, and in the form of an agreed contract. A behavioural contract covers:

- the steps to be taken if the patient fails to attend, or to meet other commitments;
- target signs, symptoms, and behaviours suggestive of possible risk or relapse;
- specific action to be taken in the event of risk or relapse;

- action to be taken in the event of a relative or carer no longer being able to provide support; and,
- the agreed plan, or the record of disagreement (in the event of a disagreement, arrangements should be made for the early involvement of a health or social services manager who is external to the CMHT, and/or a request for a second medical opinion by a Responsible Medical Officer).

## Management Options

The options for managing risk involve implementing actions designed to minimise the likelihood of future risk behaviour. These can be broadly categorised as follows:

- limiting the opportunities;
- warning potential victims;
- reducing triggers and controlling situational factors (risk factors);
- changing risk behaviour;
- monitoring and control; and,
- compulsory treatment / hospitalisation.

To illustrate these options, the following short vignettes have been included. The vignettes are based upon actual clients, although the names have been changed.

## Case Vignette No. 1: Moderate Depression with Suicide Attempts

Julie is a 23-year old woman who was initially referred by her GP to the CMHT following repeated overdoses. It transpired that Julie had made five attempts to overdose, taking anti-depressants (SSRIs) on two occasions, and paracetomol on three occasions. On three occasions, she required treatment via the Accident and Emergency Department of the local hospital and, although offered admission to a mental health unit on two occasions, she refused this. Julie had taken all of the overdoses in the last 8-month period, since being involved in a road traffic accident that caused a miscarriage. Although having recovered well from the accident, Julie had convinced herself that she would never again be able to conceive – and thus would not fulfil her dream. She reported feeling low in mood, described becoming frequently tearful, particularly if in the company of other friends with babies or young children. During the initial sessions, she again threatened to take an overdose of paracetomol, which she had obtained for the purpose. She lives with her boyfriend, whom she described as supportive, but unable to fully understand. She works as a care assistant.

*Outcomes and Issue* Julie was engaged in a short series of individual sessions by a CMHN, based upon a cognitive-behavioural approach. This incorporated problem-solving; goal-setting, both short-term and long-term; identification and reinforcement of her reasons for living as opposed to dying; disputation of unhelpful thoughts and beliefs, assisted through self-monitoring methods such as a thought record; and, addressing the issues connected with the road traffic accident and her miscarriage. Julie attended 10 sessions over a period of four months, at which point she was discharged. Whilst she threatened two further overdoses, over the course of initial sessions, she managed to maintain self-control and did not act upon such thoughts. At one-year follow-up, she had not repeated any high-risk behaviour, was engaged to be married and planning a career in health care.

Given her history of repeated overdosing, it may have been sensible to encourage an in-patient admission. However, it was reasonably decided to arrange for a period of supported community care aimed at providing Julie with a set of self-help skills, thus representing the least restrictive intervention. In view of her continued threats to overdose, this constituted a 'therapeutic risk' on the part of the clinician. Responsibility for her behaviour continued to rest with Julie. Each threat to overdose led to a further discussion of her personal goals, the likely consequences of such high-risk behaviour, reinforcing the disadvantages, and emphasising the reasons for living. She did continue to have the support of her boyfriend and family.

The options that were chosen involved Julie changing her risk behaviour as a result of the skills she acquired through engaging in a cognitive-behavioural approach. Ongoing monitoring, and the reinforcement of her self-control, was coupled with addressing the situational factors and triggers that were maintaining her distress and behaviour (the road traffic accident, the miscarriage, and the unacceptable assumption that she would never again be able to conceive). Although the CMHN was experienced, regular clinical supervision was available to help him manage the frustrations and anxieties of working with the risks presented by this client.

*Case Vignette No. 2: Avoidant Personality Disorder with Obsessive-Compulsive Features (Differential Diagnosis)*

Tony is a single, 25-year old man who first presented to mental health services about two years ago. He works as a data-entry clerk for a local bank and lives at home with his parents, two younger brothers and an older sister. He described his main problem as recurring negative thoughts about himself, which particularly happen whenever he is in the presence of other people. He reports a tendency to assume that others are thinking, will think, or say bad things about him, to the point that he prefers to avoid all social situations. Alternatively, he will instead bite his cheeks and teeth together, so as not to speak. He becomes very preoccupied with these thoughts, to the point of being very indecisive and virtually unable to achieve any action without the intervention of his mother. Tony appears very tense most of the time, and on occasions will appear very impulsive and quick. He states that this is the only way he can achieve anything because, if he stops to think, then decisions or actions become impossible. Tony describes the above as a lifelong trait, and has expressed severe frustration and hopelessness about being able to make any improvements. He has also recently been expressing suicidal ideas, of taking an overdose of paracetomol, or of jumping in front of a train. So far, he has never acted upon these ideas. He feels very stressed living at home. His mother is very protective of him and interfering; his father is quiet and passive; and, his brothers and sisters tend to criticise and demean him.

*Outcome and Issues* Following an attempt to work with Tony in the community setting and to resettle him into his own flat, he deteriorated. His mood lowered further, with almost constant preoccupation with suicidal ideas. He also expressed thoughts of self-failure, frustration, severe hopelessness and helplessness. After presenting at a community centre with paracetomol in his possession, shortly after contemplating jumping in front of a train, he was admitted to the local in-patient unit under section 3 of the *Mental Health Act* (House of Commons, 1983). Gradually, Tony began to accept the need for admission under section and began to improve.

Tony presented an unacceptable risk for continuing community care, being unable to fully engage in psychological treatment, and eventually presenting a serious and imminent risk of suicide. He had also consistently refused informal admission. He is a young man with few social contacts, who displayed severe anxiety and agitation with obsessive-compulsive features, and expressed severe hopelessness about his ability to change. He thus presented several factors, which are known to be associated with an increased risk of suicide.

The options taken involved: limiting the opportunities for a suicidal act, by admitting him to hospital; reducing the triggers / situational factors, which include social isolation (despite his family being there), and severe hopelessness; ongoing monitoring and control; and, compulsory treatment, due to his refusal of informal care.

*Case Vignette No. 3: Anti-Social Personality*

Ken is a 24-year old man recently admitted to the acute admission unit following an assault on other family members. In the unit, he is uncooperative and aggressive towards staff. If family members visit he tends towards increased aggression. There have been a couple of incidents of violence, where members of staff were injured. Ken describes considerable anxiety as his main problem, and is constantly requesting time to talk to staff about how ill he is and how things would have been different if only others had behaved differently in the past. Ken's history shows a number of significant events, in particular a period of school phobia and periods of heavy alcohol and drug use. He had been unable to keep up his job, having been dismissed for poor attendance and arguing with work-mates. In the cases where he had become violent, he believes that it was the fault of the other person(s) and that they got what they deserved. Analysis of the incidents by ward staff revealed that Ken appeared to be choosing the times and victims carefully. Violence, unless it was against his parents, would always involve staff alone in isolated parts of the Unit.

*Outcomes and Issues* - The first concern here is for the safety of all concerned. There is an obvious focus on aggression and violence towards his parents, as well as a more diffuse risk towards staff in the Unit. The 'knee-jerk' reaction from a number of those involved, was to call for his discharge. This is a mistake. Whilst it is absolutely the case that staff on wards must be able to carry out their duties safely, discharging Ken would have put his parents at risk. Short-term solutions to individual incidents might involve seclusion, medication or 2 to 1 nursing (1 to 1 nursing should never be the response to a violent patient, as it only provides a potential victim in a situation that is practically guaranteed to raise tensions anyway). The longer-term answer here was to move Ken to a local secure unit where his behaviours were more controlled, and boundaries were more clearly set. In addition, visits by his parents were supervised in order to give them more protection. Longer-term plans involved a move to a staffed hostel rather than discharge home, with visits home dependent upon his behaviour the previous week. At that stage, if Ken should go missing from the hostel, his parents would be alerted immediately. The police might also be informed if his last contact with the hostel staff gave rise to concerns that he was angry with his parents.

This case raises another significant issue. Sometimes, relatives and carers will not verbalise their real wishes for fear of upsetting the patient, or for fear of further aggression. Professionals need, firstly, to give the opportunity for carers to speak without the knowledge of the patient. Secondly, they should be prepared to overrule the stated wishes of carers, if the multi-disciplinary team feels that the carers are putting themselves at longer-term risk.

*Case Vignette No. 4*: *Command Hallucinations and Self-Neglect*

Wilma is a 38-year old woman who had recently moved into the CMHT's catchment area. She lives with her husband who has had to give up work in order to care for her. At initial assessment, he describes never being able to leave her alone for fear of what she might do. The couple have no children, and Wilma very much wants to be a mother. Wilma would remain in bed all day and eat little or nothing if it wasn't for her husband's encouragement. The worrying feature is that she hears two different voices: one tells her to harm herself, and one tells her to steal a baby from a pram. Her husband stated that he had on many occasions stopped her from taking knives from the kitchen drawer, and had to hide her medication because she had taken small overdoses in the past. He also mentioned that once, while out shopping, he had been forced to physically remove her from the vicinity of a pram after she had tried to pick up the baby. Wilma admitted later that she was hearing the voice telling her to steal the baby at that time. The house they live in is in a small row of four terraced houses in an isolated location. They do not have a car, but could reach the local town on the infrequent bus service.

*Outcomes and Issues* - The immediate concerns in this case are risk to children and to Wilma. There is also the risk of self-neglect. The key to all the above is the fact that the husband is remaining at home with Wilma, and made it clear that he never leaves her. The presence of command hallucinations that have been acted on makes the risk of self-harm or stealing a baby high. Despite this, the members of the team that assessed Wilma were happy for her to remain at home as long as her husband continued with his commitment. Because of the isolated location of the house, it was felt that even if Wilma should leave the house alone, there would be time to put the management plan into operation . The husband has the most important role here, as he will need to inform the authorities should he lose track of Wilma. Because of this, the team members also carried out an assessment of the husband's capacity to understand the issues at stake and make the needed decisions. It was agreed that he would be unlikely to fail in this. If he lost track of his wife he was to inform the CMHT and the police as soon as possible. It would also be necessary to have some contact with the police about this matter. This could be handled in a number of ways, depending on the relationship between the team and their local force, and on the perceived risk presented. The first option is to approach them only if the team loses contact with Wilma. Other options include: informing the police straight away and asking them to contact the team if there is a missing baby (without revealing the name of the client), or telling the police the identity of the person the team is worried about. The latter option would produce the quickest response, but would mean revealing information about the client that could be construed as a breach of confidentiality, given that no crime has been committed. If the client had had previous convictions for stealing babies and lived alone, the latter options would be the only ones to consider.

The other components of the plan involve twice weekly visits to Wilma to monitor the situation; referring Wilma and her husband to the local Befrienders service, to reduce their isolation; and, arranging respite care for Wilma so that the situation does not become too much for the husband.

*Further Practical Considerations for Management*

It is essential that part of the management plan for both violence and suicide is the inclusion of therapeutic activity. This should be aimed at undermining the reasons for the undesirable behaviour, and boosting reasons for more acceptable behaviour. Cognitive Behaviour Therapy (CBT) offers a number of approaches that can be effective for this (Persons, 1989).

## Concluding Discussion

### Risk Management

Conducting a comprehensive risk assessment is only part of the task facing CMHNs. Next, it is necessary to develop a management plan. This, as might be expected, should detail the actions to be carried out in order to minimise the risk. We choose the word 'minimise' deliberately, as we feel that eliminating risk is what is aimed for, but never achieved in an absolute sense. It must, therefore, be part of the process of risk management to assess the extent to which an intervention will reduce the risk. This has to be balanced against availability of, and demand on, resources. For example, to what extent does a CMHN visiting a client three times per week reduce risk of suicide in comparison with one visit per week? Obviously, the client's individual circumstances will have great bearing on this. However, if the CMHN was carrying out a course of CBT designed to challenge the client's suicidal ideation, it is likely to have more value than more frequent visits 'just' to check on the client's mental state. The other message here is that risk reduction is not solely about controlling the client, but is also about treatment of the problem.

For a risk management plan to be effective, it should not only say what everyone involved should do, but must also spell out the 'what ifs ?'. The fear of what might happen will have been established from the assessment. Therefore, it needs to be decided what would constitute an indicator of the likelihood that any of these behaviours were increasing, or have already happened. Following that, a plan should be made of the action that needs to be taken in the event of any of the indicators occurring.

### Dilemma of Risk Management

One of the dilemmas of a risk management system is the balance between usability and completeness. The system needs to be as simple as possible to avoid errors. It also needs to be practical within services that are, by and large, very busy and often short of staff. On the other hand, gathering more information increases the likelihood that the professional's decision-making will be better informed. There is no perfect answer to this challenge. Nevertheless, we do have a suggestion of a way to reduce the problem. Risk assessment protocols should be layered so that everyone contacting services gets a low-level assessment that is gathered from the usual clinical assessment carried out in the service. Where that indicates the possibility of increased risk, a more in-depth risk assessment is carried out. This concentrates the effort on those with greatest need, and reduces the overall workload for the service.

*Communication*

One of the single most important factors in the team management of risk is communication. As mentioned above, one only has to read the reports of any of the recent inquiries into serious incidents to see that poor communication can undermine the best of plans. It is vital that information should be passed on to all those who need to know. This can cause difficulties because of the tension between communication and confidentiality. When it comes to life being at risk, the issue of confidentiality is something of a 'red herring'. There is no excuse for not passing information to any individual who may be at risk from not knowing. This extends beyond health and social care staff, to include anyone having contact with the client. It would be foolish to have CMHNs visit a client in pairs if, an hour after they have left, the housing officer or the client's GP arrives on their own.

There is often reluctance to involve the police in plans to manage risk, but they are very much part of the process. In reality, if organisations can foster good relationships with the local police force, it can lead to far more effective help for clients. For example, earlier involvement of mental health clinicians may be achieved following an incident, or after being informed by an officer that a client with a history of suicide has been seen late at night on the canal tow path. There is, of course, one over-riding reason why good communication is vital. If the risks are not known, then it is not possible to provide the right services for the client and, as a result of that, their care suffers.

It is perhaps obvious that communication must be understandable, and yet many practitioners will use language that others do not understand.

Medical terminology in particular may not mean anything to many of those involved in the care of the client. Therefore, risks and the management of those risks, must be described plainly and simply. A further point here is that descriptions should be as comprehensive and as detailed as possible, in order to inform decision-making. For example: 'This man has three convictions for ABH' means far less than: 'This man has three convictions for ABH against his mother'. In turn, that is less useful than: 'This man has three convictions for ABH against his mother, all of which happened when he had been drinking heavily'. Hopefully, it is easier to construct a management plan from the latter description.

Access to the information is also crucial. Many long-term patients of mental health services have a great deal of risk information buried in a 5-inch thick folder of notes (if you are lucky). This information is not held in a useful form. It is necessary for all services to have a method for keeping risk information together in a form that is easy to access. Probably the best system is an electronic record on a networked computer system. Paper records can also achieve this aim, but it is important that, as patients move around services, new records are not started. Otherwise, there will be confusion about which is the real risk management plan.

## Multi-Agency Working

The difficulties of multi-agency working are well known. Many inquiries have identified problems, and the main reason for introducing the CPA was to attempt to overcome the difficulties. The agencies most frequently working together are health and social services, but many other agencies might be involved, for example, the criminal justice agencies, voluntary organisations, local authorities and others.

Agencies that often work together must get together and draw up joint policies and procedures. It is not sufficient just to have a joint understanding of CPA. Risk assessment must also be the same. Often the mistake can be made of thinking that using the same forms means that agencies are working together. This will not be so until the organisations involved also have a shared understanding of the meaning of risk assessment, as well as a shared understanding of each agency's role in the management of that risk. This is best achieved with joint training to complement the common paperwork and policies.

## Case Against Admission

Often the first response to an identified suicide risk is to seek admission to an in-patient facility. This can be a mistake. That first reaction is usually prompted by the wish to preserve the client's safety. But acute in-patient units are never completely safe places to be, unless the client is placed on continuous observation. For many clients, it is possible that the quality of intervention may decrease if the ward they go to is consistently busy or under-staffed. If there is good social support from relatives and friends, coupled with an effective treatment (whether that be medical or psychological), it may well be better to keep the client at home. The reality is that they may get more support that way. There is also the possibility that being hospitalised may seem to the client to be proof of their failure, and hence lead to an increase in risk.

## Clinical Supervision: Coping with Risk

As stated within the guidelines for the local Trust (Butler and Suppiah, 1996, p. 1), supervision may be:

> viewed as a structured, on-going and objective process in which a more experienced peer or more senior person maintains a negotiated contractual relationship with the individual nurse, assisting him/her to focus and reflect upon his/her professional role and clinical practice, thereby facilitating professional development. In order for supervision to be effective, it should be well-structured, uninterrupted and regular, each session being based upon a clear agenda agreed between supervisor and supervisee.

The guidelines describe a model for the basis of supervision, based upon three distinct and inter-related areas (Hawkins and Shohet, 1990): educative, supportive, and managerial.

Clinical supervision is viewed as helpful for both the staff member and for client care when there are issues of risk. This has been shown in a local audit study of clinical supervision across acute and community mental health teams in South Bedfordshire (Butler, 1999). Feeling supported (74%), stronger working relationships (63%) and gaining additional clinical insight (61%), were the most commonly reported outcomes of supervision in that study. Therefore, it is strongly recommended that systems for support and supervision are in place for those staff or therapists working with clients who present significant risk behaviours.

*Summary of Principles for Good Practice*

The principles of good practice in risk assessment and risk management involve the completion of *comprehensive* assessments, developed *collaboratively* and *communicated* to all those who need to know via *user-friendly* documentation. Assessment must be undertaken as an *ongoing* process if we are to ensure the implementation of *up-to-date* and *meaningful* risk management plans.

## References

Alberg, C., Hatfield, B. and Huxley, P. (eds) (1996), *Learning Materials on Mental Health: Risk Assessment*, University of Manchester / Department of Health, Manchester.

Appleby, L., Shaw, J., Amos, T., McDonnell, R., Harris, C., McCann, K., Kiernan, K., Davies, S., Bickley, H. and Parsons, R. (1999), 'Suicide Within 12-months of Contact with Mental Health Services: National Clinical Survey', *British Medical Journal*, vol. 318, pp. 1235-9 .

Beck, A.T. (1967), *Depression: Causes and Treatment*, University of Philadelphia, Philadelphia.

Beck, A.T. (1986), 'Hopelessness as a Predictor of Eventual Suicide', in J.J. Mann and M. Stanley (eds), *Psychobiology*, Academy of Sciences, New York.

Beck, A.T. and Steer, R.A. (1988), *Manual for Beck Hopelessness Scale*, Psychological Corporation., San Antonio.

Beck, A.T., Steer, R.A. and Ranieri, W.F. (1988), 'Scale for Suicide Ideation: Psychometric Properties of a Self-Report Version', *Journal of Clinical Psychology*, vol. 44, pp. 499-505.

Beck, A.T., Ward, C.H., Mendelson, M., Mock, J. and Erbaugh, J. (1961), 'An Inventory for Measuring Depression', *Archives of General Psychiatry*, vol. 4, pp. 561-71.

Beck, A.T., Weissman, A. and Kovacs, J. (1976), 'Alcoholism, Hopelessness and Suicidal Behaviour', *Journal of Studies on Alcohol*, vol. 37, pp. 66-77.

Beck, A.T., Weissman, A., Lester, D. and Trexler, L. (1974), 'The Measurement of Pessimism: The Hopelessness Scale', *Journal of Consulting and Clinical Psychology*, vol. 42, pp. 861-5.

Blom-Cooper, L., Hally, H. and Murphy, E. (1995), *The Falling Shadow – One Patient's Mental Health Care, 1978-93*, Duckworth and Co., London.

Borum, R. (1996), 'Improving the Clinical Practice of Violence Risk Assessment: Technology, Guidelines and Training', *American Psychologist*, vol. 51(9), pp. 945-56.

Bourget, D. and Bradford, J.M.W. (1990), 'Homicidal Parents', *Canadian Journal of Psychiatry*, vol 35, pp. 233-7.

British Psychological Society (1997a), *A CORE (Centre for Clinical Outcomes, Research and Effectiveness) Assessment and Outcomes Package for the Care Programme Approach*, University College London, London.

British Psychological Society (1997b), *CORE Risk Assessment Manual and Risk Profile*, University College London, London.

Butler, J. (1999), 'Clinical Supervision: Developing, Implementing and Evaluating Practice Standards in Acute and Community Mental Health', *South Bedfordshire Community Health Care Trust Journal of Clinical Practice*, vol. 1(4), pp. 96-102.

Butler, J. and Suppiah, V. (1996), *Guidelines on Clinical Supervision for Nursing Staff*, South Bedfordshire Community Health Care Trust, Luton.

Campion, J.F., Cravens, J.M. and Covan, F. (1988), 'A Study of Filicidal Men', *American Journal of Psychiatry*, vol. 145, no. 9, pp. 1141-4.

Clark, D.C. and Fawcett, J. (1992), 'Review of Empirical Risk Factors for Evaluation of the Suicidal Patient', in R. Bongor (ed), *Suicide*, Oxford University Press, Oxford, chapter 2.

Crichton, J. (1995), 'A Review of Psychiatric In-patient Violence', in J. Crichton, *Psychiatric Patient Violence*, Duckworth and Co., London.

Department of Health (1999), *A National Service Framework for Mental Health: Modern Standards and Service Models*, Department of Health, London.

Dyer, J.A.T. and Kreitman, N. (1984), 'Hopelessness, Depression and Suicidal Intent in Parasuicide', *British Journal of Psychiatry*, vol. 144, pp. 127-33.

Eldrid, J., (1988), *Caring for the Suicidal*, Constable, London.

Fairlie, A. and Butler, J. (1994), *Suicides in Bedfordshire: 1991 and 1992*, South Bedfordshire Community Health Care Trust, Luton.

Hawkins, P. and Shohet, R. (1990), *Supervision in the Helping Professions*, Oxford University Press, Milton Keynes.

Hawton, K. (1987), 'Assessment of Suicide Risk', *British Journal of Psychiatry*, vol. 150, pp. 145-53.

Hawton, K. and Catalan, J. (1987), *Assessment of Suicide Risk in Attempted Suicide*, Oxford University Press, Oxford.

Hawton, K. and Fagg, J. (1988), 'Suicides and Other Causes of Death Following Attempted Suicide', *British Journal of Psychiatry*, vol. 152, pp. 259-66.

House of Commons (1983), *The Mental Health Act*, HMSO, London.

Kemshall, H. (1999), 'Risk Assessment and Risk Management: Practice and Policy Implications', *British Journal of Forensic Practice*, vol. 1, pp. 27-36.

Kreitman, N. (ed) (1977), *Parasuicide*, John Wiley, Chichester.

Kreitman, N. (1987), in C. Sutton, *Handbook of Research for Helping Professions*, Royal College of Psychiatrists, London.

Kreitman, N. and Dyer, J.A.T. (1980), 'Suicide in Relation to Parasuicide', *Medical Education*, pp. 1827-30.

Lidz, C.W., Mulvey, P. and Gardner, W. (1993), 'The Accuracy of Predictions of Violence to Others', *Journal of American Medical Association*, vol. 269(8), pp. 1007-11.

Lipsedge, M. and Bland, S.R. (1997), 'Review of 11 Independent Inquiries into Homicides by Psychiatric Patients', *Clinical Risk*, vol. 3, pp. 171-77.

Main, J., Wilkins, J., Pope, D. and Manikon, S. (1996), *The Report of the Independent Inquiry Team into the Care and Treatment of Nilesh Gadher*, Ealing, Hammersmith and Hounslow Health Authority, London.

McClure, G.M.G. (1984), 'Suicide in England and Wales, 1975-84', *British Journal of Psychiatry*, vol. 144, pp. 119-26.

McLaughlin, C. (1993), 'Suicidal Behaviour', *British Journal of Nursing*, vol. 2, no. 22, pp. 1103-5.

Mishcon, J., Dick, D., Milne, I., Beard, P. and Mackay, J. (1996), *The Hampshire Report: Report of the Independent Inquiry Team into the Care and Treatment of Francis Hampshire*, Redbridge and Waltham Forest Health Authority, Essex.

Morgan, H. (1979), *Death Wishes? The Understanding and Management of Deliberate Self-Harm*, John Wiley, Chichester.

Persons, J.B. (1989), *Cognitive Therapy in Practice: A Case Formulation Approach*, Norton, London.

Prins, H.A. (1981), 'Dangerous People or Dangerous Situations? Some Implications for Assessment and Management', *Medical Science and Law*, vol. 21(2), pp. 125-33.

Ritchie, J.H., Dick, D. and Lingham, R. (1994), *The Report of the Inquiry into the Care and Treatment of Christopher Clunis*, HMSO, London.

Sainsbury, P. (1955), 'Suicide in London', *Maudsley Monograph No. 1*, Chapman and Hall, London.

South Bedfordshire Community Health Care Trust (1998), *Community Care Policy for People Receiving Care from Mental Health Services*, South Bedfordshire Community Mental Health Care, Luton.

Schneidman, E.S. (ed) (1976), *Suicide Notes Reconsidered in Suicidology: Contemporary Developments*, Grune and Stratton, New York.

Steadman, H.J., Monahan, J., Appelbaum, P.S., Grisso, T., Mulvey, E.P., Roth, L.H., Robbins, P.C. and Klassen, D. (1994), 'Designing a New Generation of Risk Assessment Research', in J. Monahan and H.J. Steadman (eds), *Violence and Mental Disorder: Developments in Risk Assessment*, University of Chicago, Chicago / London.

Swanson, J.W., Holzer, C.E., Ganju, V.K. and Jones, R.T. (1990), 'Violence and Psychiatric Disorder in the Community: Evidence from the Epidemiologic

Catchment Area Surveys', *Hospital and Community Psychiatry*, vol. 41, pp. 761-70.

Tardiff, K. and Sweillam, J. (1980), 'Assault, Suicide, Mental Illness', *Archives of General Psychiatry,* vol. 37, pp.164-9.

Tuckman, J. and Youngman, W.F. (1963), 'Identifying Suicide Risk Groups among Attempted Suicides', *Public Health Reports*, vol. 78, pp. 763-6.

Tuckman, J. and Youngman, W.F. (1968), 'A Scale for Assessing Suicide Risk of Attempted Suicides', *Journal of Clinical Psychology*, vol. 24, pp. 17-19.

Webster, C.D., Eaves, D., Douglas, K. and Wintrup, A. (1995), *The HCR-20 Scheme: The Assessment of Dangerousness and Risk,* Simon Fraser University and Psychiatric Services Commission of British Columbia, Burnaby, British Columbia.

Whitlock, F. (1973), 'Suicide in England and Wales, 1959-63', *Psychological Medicine*, vol. 3, pp. 350-65; 411-20.